DIABETES NO MORE

DR. BHUJANG SHETTY

STARDOM BOOKS

www.StardomBooks.com

STARDOM BOOKS, LLC
112, Bordeaux Ct,
Coppell, TX 75019

FIRST EDITION OCTOBER 2023

STARDOM BOOKS

A Division of Stardom Alliance
112, Bordeaux Ct,
Coppell, TX 75019

www.stardombooks.com

Stardom Books, United States
Stardom Books, India

DIABETES NO MORE

Dr. Bhujang Shetty

p. 300
cm. 13.5 X 21.5

Category:
CKB025000 - Cooking: Health & Healing - Diabetic
& Sugar Free
HEA039050 - Health & Fitness: Diseases - Diabetes

ISBN: 978-1-957456-20-1

DEDICATION

This book is dedicated to my parents.

CONTENTS

ACKNOWLEDGMENTS

I would like to offer my gratitude to Dr. Stephen Phineey, Dr. Benjamin Bikman, Dr. Paul Mason, Prof. Tim Noakes, Dr. Gary Fettke, Dr. Jeff Volek, Prof. Robert Lustig, Dr. Peter Brunker, Dr. Bret Scher, Dr. Ken D Berry, Dr. David Unwin, Dr. Sten Ekberg, and Dr. Eric Berg for their contributions to the field of health and nutrition. What I have learned from each of their work forms the core of this book. I would also like to acknowledge the impact Sadhguru, Deepak Chopra, Eckhart Tolle, and Sister Shivani have had on me over the years. Their teachings have made me introspect and lead a better life.

I offer my profound thanks to Dr. Chaitra Jayadev for her work and contribution. I am grateful for the time and effort she has taken to help me complete the book. I would also like to express my gratitude to Dr. Anand Vinekar for his contributions. I thank Dr. Major Narendra for travelling along with me on this journey.
I extend my gratitude to our institute's multimedia team for designing the creative illustrations. I thank Mrs. Chitra Seshadri, Mrs. Shubha Iyengar, Mr. Abdul Muthalib, Mrs. Shilpa Rudra and all the doctors and staff of Narayana Nethralaya for their support.

I must thank my patients for having faith in me and inspiring me to get started on this book. I am indebted to my family members for standing by me and encouraging me to write this book. I thank my son, Dr. Naren Shetty, for helping me design the cover page. Contributions for the Recipes by Mrs. Pushpa Krishnappa, Prof. Krishnappa, Mrs. Ashwini K Chakrasali, Mrs. Navitha Reddy and RDC Team is gratefully acknowledged.

If any material reproduced has not been duly acknowledged, please accept my sincere apologies.

Finally, I am grateful to Raam Anand and the team at Stardom Books for helping me turn this book into a reality.

The author was a medical doctor and has used scientifically researched and evidence-based methods to substantiate what he has written. The thoughts expressed are based on his personal experiences of attempting, modifying, relearning and then teaching. The contents of this book must not be considered as medical advice.

INTRODUCTION

"People are fed by the food industry, which pays no attention to health; and are treated by the health industry, which pays no attention to food."
— *Wendell Berry*

It was only 50 years ago that most societies consumed plenty of saturated fat in butter, milk, cream, and fatty meats. Later, based on some poorly conducted research, we were convinced that fatty food leads to obesity and fat-clogged arteries, resulting in various heart-related diseases.

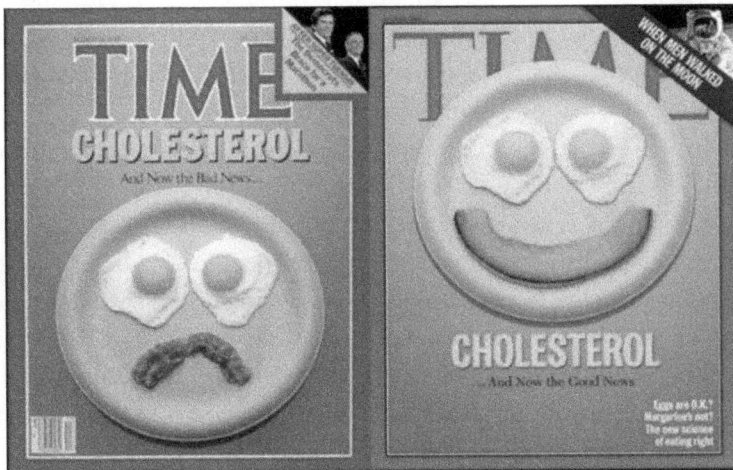

Fig. 1: An indication of how 'Time' has changed our thinking

So, it was recommended to switch to a low-fat diet and its associated guidelines in the form of a food pyramid. However, this switch to a low-fat diet resulted in an increased carbohydrate intake of grains, cereals, bread, and rice. Additionally, manufacturers replaced the fat in many "low fat" foods with sugars to improve the taste. The incidence of obesity and Type 2 diabetes has steadily increased with this change in dietary habits, owing to the excess carbohydrates rather than excess fat. According to evidence in the book "The Schwarzbein Principle," putting pre-diabetic patients on a low-fat, high-carb diet created an increased development of diabetes. On the other hand, a low-carb, high and healthy-fat diet with moderate proteins successfully reverses diabetes. This was established in 1850, even before we knew what insulin was or how it worked in the body. It was proved that you could reverse diabetes with low carbs, and that you can also lose weight with low carbohydrate.

We are so used to hearing that we are supposed to eat a low-fat and high-carb diet, that we have developed a fat phobia. Whenever we eat sugar or carbs, they are broken down into their simplest form – glucose – in the gut and absorbed into the bloodstream. To keep the blood glucose levels down, the body produces a hormone known as insulin (in the pancreas) to take the sugar out of the blood and put it into the cell to be used as energy. The cell uses whatever it needs and converts the rest of the sugar into fat.

Insulin is a fat storing hormone, and insulin resistance (which is pre-diabetes) develops only in response to high sugars and carbohydrates. It not only stores fat but also locks it up! When you eat more sugar, your insulin stays high, and the insulin tells the cell to hold on to the fats. As long as you have high insulin, there is no way for your body to retrieve that fat and use it for energy. Although your body is supposed to have a balance between fat storing and fat burning, when your insulin is high, the preference is to store the fat. This can make you hungry because you have no access to the energy stored as fat. While carbs increase your blood sugar, fats, on the other hand, do not stimulate insulin nor create a lot of volatility in your blood sugar.

So, start reducing the carbs over a period of time to reduce that insulin resistance. Another thing that you want to keep in mind is that regular exercise is a simple way to reduce insulin resistance. Making your muscles work makes them more sensitive to insulin. There is a physiological change in the receptors - it will take in more blood sugar with less insulin.

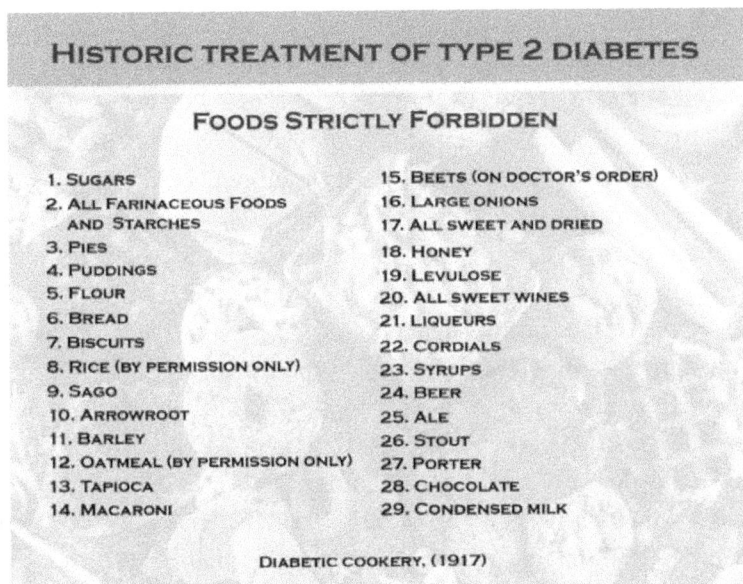

HISTORIC TREATMENT OF TYPE 2 DIABETES

FOODS STRICTLY FORBIDDEN

1. SUGARS	15. BEETS (ON DOCTOR'S ORDER)
2. ALL FARINACEOUS FOODS AND STARCHES	16. LARGE ONIONS
	17. ALL SWEET AND DRIED
3. PIES	18. HONEY
4. PUDDINGS	19. LEVULOSE
5. FLOUR	20. ALL SWEET WINES
6. BREAD	21. LIQUEURS
7. BISCUITS	22. CORDIALS
8. RICE (BY PERMISSION ONLY)	23. SYRUPS
9. SAGO	24. BEER
10. ARROWROOT	25. ALE
11. BARLEY	26. STOUT
12. OATMEAL (BY PERMISSION ONLY)	27. PORTER
13. TAPIOCA	28. CHOCOLATE
14. MACARONI	29. CONDENSED MILK

DIABETIC COOKERY. (1917)

Fig. 2: Forbidden foods for diabetics as advised in 1917

One classic sign of insulin resistance is getting tired after eating a meal. This is because your body cannot process it properly, and the blood sugar shoots up. Then your body has to expend a lot of energy to convert that blood sugar into triglycerides or fat. While this is one sign, people can have many different presentations, and many people can have what we call a 'roller-coaster' of blood sugar levels. Another sign is irritability, or the inability to go on for several hours without a meal. Your body is designed to have a stable level of blood sugar, and when you don't eat, it has mechanisms to maintain blood sugar levels from stores of fats and glycogen.

But when your body cannot do that, you get irritable, hungry, lightheaded, or develop headaches.

If you feel like you have to eat something every two to three hours - you probably have insulin resistance along with high blood sugar levels. This is because you have taught your body to rely solely on sugar or carbohydrates for energy. When you rely only on sugar, you increase your insulin levels and cannot pull energy out of your fat stores. So, your body doesn't have a backup for energy, and that is why you have to keep eating all that food. You depend on all those snacks, primarily sugar and carbs, because that's what your body has learned to live off.

Most young people metabolize carbohydrates quite well, but over time, especially when exposed to large amounts of carbs, many become insulin-resistant. In other words, insulin becomes less effective because blood sugars are elevated (Type 2 diabetes) and obesity develops. A diet low in carbohydrates and high in "good" fats is very effective in weight loss. There is also evidence that it reduces the likelihood of developing Type 2 diabetes, fatty liver and possibly other diseases such as dementia, Alzheimer's disease and some forms of cancer. So, it makes sense to reduce carbohydrate intake. At the same time, it is important to replace carbohydrates with an alternative energy source – healthy fats. Fat has been unnecessarily demonized over recent years, but there is no scientific evidence that high-quality fat causes any kind of disease, particularly cardiovascular disease. However, there are good fats and bad fats. Good fats such as butter, extra-virgin olive oil, and coconut oil are natural fats and will not harm you. On the other hand, trans-fats found in processed and hydrogenated vegetable oils are not good fats because they are full of toxins due to the harsh processing and should be avoided.

Once your body develops a habit and depends on something, it will not give it up without a little bit of a fight. But it is not as difficult as you think. So, move away from the carbs gradually and start replacing it with healthy fat in your diet. Before you know it, you will find that you have a little bit more stability. A high-fat diet gives satiety and reduces hunger and cravings. Hence, one will be able to go six to eight hours without feeling weak or irritable.

Your physiology is the same as your ancestors, and they did not wake up to tea or have a breakfast buffet. They had to go out and hunt or gather food. Hunter-gatherer tribes to this day have to go out and find or catch something before they can eat, and that's what your physiology is adapted to.

We feed our pets once or twice a day and not every two hours because they are adapted to their food supply. In nature, it works even better because animals don't eat things out of a can. You can start with reducing the worst carbs first - what we call the white trash - the white flour and the white sugar.

Even with minimal carb intake and in the absence of glucose, the body can maintain sufficient blood glucose for the brain through a process called gluconeogenesis. It has also been shown that the brain can function perfectly well using ketone bodies as its primary energy source. While fatty acids are essential and amino acids from protein are essential, there is no such thing as essential carbohydrates. You can live for years and years without a single gram of carbohydrate and still do really well without developing diabetes or heart disease. Look at the Eskimos who do it all the time. You don't have to worry about eating zero carbs because almost everything has a little bit of carbs. Your spinach, lettuce, cauliflower, and broccoli, all have carbohydrates. This is the best form of carbohydrate because it is not a grain and it is fibrous and water-rich, and because it is absorbed infinitely slowly, it has virtually no impact on insulin. That is why these carbs have a very low glycemic index. With that brief overview, let us look at each of these components of getting healthy and reversing diabetes more in detail in the subsequent chapters.

"It's unfortunate that your bad diet won't allow you to live and your good doctor won't allow you to die. Between your bad diet and the good doctor, you are tortured to death."

DR. BHUJANG SHETTY

PART A:
FOOD AND YOUR HEALTH

1

MY STORY

Now that you know why I set out to write this book and what I plan to convey, let's begin with my story: I was born in 1953 and was diagnosed with diabetes at the age of 40. Diabetes is a disease that runs in my family. Therefore, this wasn't much of a shock, but the disease hit me just during the period when I was trying to find my feet in my professional career.

The stress of establishing an eye hospital and my genetic predisposition may have fueled the fire. My physician put me on tablets, asked me to avoid sweets, and exercise regularly. This is the typical advice given to all diabetic patients.

Days passed and with time, the number of tablets I had to consume also increased. I had no option but to follow the treatment to keep my blood sugar levels stable. Diabetes exposed me to a wide range of accompanied complications like high cholesterol, heart-related disorders, kidney issues, bladder problems and much more.

The situation worsened to the point when a dozen tablets were needed every day to keep all these complications under control.

	Nov 2018	Jan 2022
Weight	78.90 kg	68.75 kg
BMI	26.4	23.2
Body fat	23.8%	19.4%
Fat-free Body weight	60.12 kg	55.40 kg
Subcutaneous Fat	21.0%	17.3%
Visceral Fat	9	6
Body Water	55.0%	58.2%
Skeletal Muscle	49.2%	52.1%
Muscle Mass	57.1kg	52.60kg
Bone Mass	3.0kg	2.77kg
Protein	17.4%	18.4%
BMR	1668kcal	1566kcal
Metabolic Age	65	64

Fig. 3: Reversing my metabolic age in my health journey

At the beginning of 2021, after much research, I started a low carbohydrate, healthy fat diet (LCHF). To my surprise, within three weeks of the change, my blood sugar levels dropped and I could reduce my diabetes tablets. My blood test reports also revealed that my triglyceride levels were returning to the normal range. Through this book, I intend to share with you all my learnings. I will tell you how I completely reversed my diabetes and stopped all my medications for high cholesterol, heart and kidney issues. Please read ahead and also do your own research with due diligence. If you are convinced, try the right food practices as a remedy to all your health problems, just like I did.

	BEFORE LCHF WITH MEDICINE Jan 2021	AFTER LCHF WITHOUT MEDICINE Nov 2021
Weight	80 kg	70 kg
HbA1c	7.3%	6.3%
Triglycerides (Bad cholesterol)	330 mg/dL	110 mg/dL
HDL Cholesterol (Good cholesterol)	35 mg/dL	55 mg/dL
SGOT SGPT (Fatty liver parameters)	74 U/L (Fatty liver) 101 U/L	18 U/L (Normal liver) 16 U/L
Prostrate (in gm)	65 gm	60 gm
Serum creatinine	1.40 mg/dL	1.10 mg/dL

Fig. 4: Improvement in my health parameters after starting a low carbohydrate, healthy fat diet.

A piece of advice: If you are under medication for any health issues, it is best to seek professional guidance before reducing or stopping your medicines.

"When we got independence, our life expectancy was around 35 years, now it has doubled to almost 70 years. Though our life expectancy has grown, our health expectancy has not."

2

OUR HEALTH IS IN
OUR HANDS

"We cannot change what we are not aware of, and once we are aware, we cannot help but change."
— Sheryl Sandberg

Health is the biggest wealth in life. But, most of us often forget this, thanks to our busy lifestyle. Just like the value of water is recognized only when the well dries up, humans also realize the importance of good health only when they fall sick. According to reports from the *Center For Science in the Public Interest*, an unhealthy diet led to about 6,78,000 deaths annually in the U.S; if we don't take good care of it, our body will eventually give up on us. Health and happiness are paramount and we should prioritize them. There are some things that money can't buy – good health is one of them.

Evolution of man has been a lengthy process during which we originated from ape-like ancestors and evolved into our present-day form. This change in our physical characteristics happened gradually over several million years and several generations.

However, indulging in a sedentary lifestyle and bad food habits in the last 40 years has caused our body to undergo a rapid change from "fit to flab" within a short span of time. As a result, we have become the victims of this change and ended up developing obesity, metabolic syndrome, diabetes, heart disease, and stroke.

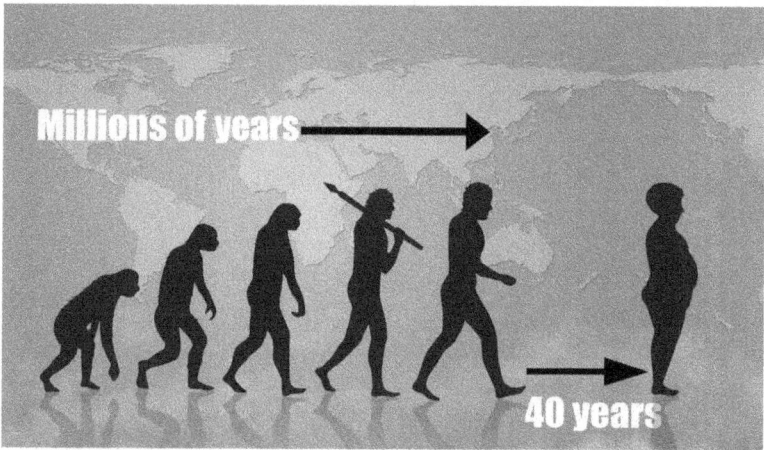

Fig. 5: Timeline Evolution from an ape to a man compared to evolution from a fit man to an obese man

Who is your partner for life? Your mom, dad, wife, husband, son, daughter, or friends?
No! None of them!
Your real-life partner is your body.
Once your body stops responding, you have no one…
You and your body stay together from birth until death.
What you do to your body is your responsibility.
The condition of your body reflects the sum of your actions.
The more you care for your body, the more your body will care for you.

What you eat, what you do to be fit, how you deal with stress, how much rest you give your body… All this will decide how your body is going to respond. Remember, your body is your responsibility, and nobody else can shoulder this burden for you. YOU yourself are your real-life partner. Take care of yourself and be fit. Money comes and goes, so do relatives and friends. No one can help you but yourself.

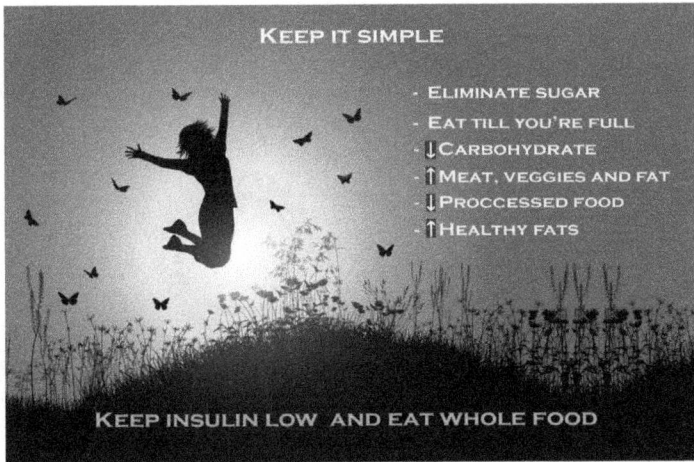

Fig 6: Foods to eat and those to avoid

While good health is a blessing, bad health can be your worst nightmare when things go wrong! So, adopt a good and healthy diet that keeps you sound, both physically and mentally. Here is an interesting thought: If we place a bunch of bananas before a monkey on one side and a bundle of cash on the other, the monkey will choose the bananas. It does not know that money can buy a lot more bananas than it is being offered. Similarly, if humans had to choose between money and health, they are most likely to choose money because they don't realize that with good health, they can earn more money and be happier in the long run! Human beings often tend to give in to temptation and take wrong decisions. We should remember that this is our body and that we are solely responsible for how it turns out. Our health is in our hands.

"It is very sad that the scientific community cannot come to a consensus regarding what constitutes a healthy diet. They are causing more confusion than ever because each one is defending their recommendation like a religion."

3

OUR BODY IS A HYBRID MACHINE

*"Your body is an incredibly intelligent machine,
you need to fuel it with the right fuel."*

Within our bodies, there are millions of chemical reactions happening all the time. The sum or the combination of all of these reactions is what we call metabolism. If these reactions are more active, then your metabolic rate is high. If there are fewer reactions, then your metabolic rate is lower. Suffice to say, whatever is happening in the body needs energy to get that work done. In order to get energy, we must eat. The three macronutrients in our diet are carbohydrates, proteins, and fats. Two of these are primarily used as fuel - carbohydrates and fat. Whether we use fat or carbohydrate depends on insulin, which is a hormone that flows through our blood and determines what energy the body is using. Since insulin determines what kind of energy we use, let's see what happens to insulin levels when we eat. When one eats pure carbohydrates like bread, cereal, or rice, there is a substantial increase in insulin, even ten times higher than normal, and it can stay elevated for up to four hours. In contrast, if someone consumes fat in their diet, there is a negligible effect on insulin.

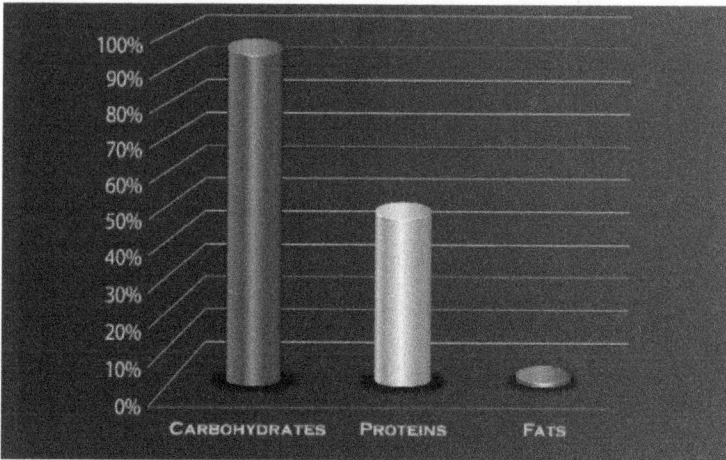

Fig. 7: *Effect on insulin release by each of the macronutrients.*

When insulin is elevated, the body starts to use or get more of its energy from carbohydrates. Basically, the body goes into a sugar burning mode. In contrast, if insulin levels are low, the body starts to burn more fat for fuel. Like the engine of a hybrid car that can use two types of fuel, the body can switch its energy source depending on the insulin levels, which is dependent on the carb intake. This concept of being able to switch between fuel sources is called metabolic flexibility. We need this flexibility to be healthy. The metabolic engine in our body is able to switch between these two fuel sources. If it is not getting any or very low carbs (less than 10% of the total energy intake), only then can it burn fat for fuel.

If we are burning more sugar, it means that we are burning less fat. And if we are not burning fat, then the amount of fat that we have in our body naturally goes up.

The solution is quite simple - if we have more fat than we want in our body and if we want to burn this fat, we have to use the fat for fuel. This will only be possible if we lower the carbohydrate intake to allow the fat we have stored to become the main energy source for the body. This will ensure that our fat tissue starts to shrink.

Unfortunately, what ends up happening is that we eat so much refined starch and sugar that it pushes the insulin levels up. The body gets stuck in a sugar-burning mode because insulin is chronically elevated. We do not let our bodies switch to burning fat for fuel and the fat levels in the body start to climb. This situation, where the body cannot switch to fat-burning is known as metabolic inflexibility.

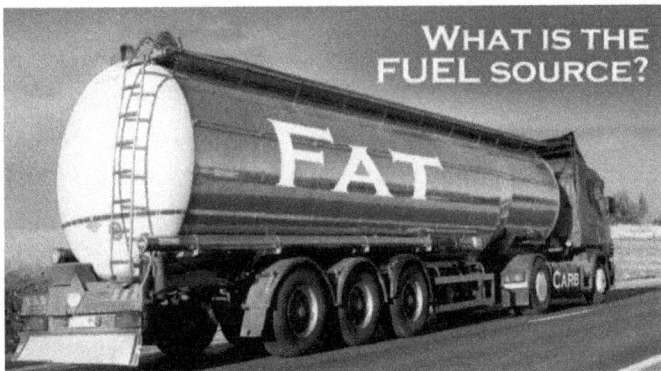

Fig. 8: Metabolic flexibility to switch between fuel sources

Metabolic flexibility had subtly but diligently served us throughout history in times of surplus when food was plentiful and in times of famine when food was scarce. However, today, because of the way we eat, most of us find ourselves with surplus energy, perpetually. We have become better at storing energy than using energy. This reality has changed the way our bodies function, leading to an astronomical increase in poor metabolic health around the world. So how do we stop it? After consuming carbohydrates, our bodies convert that food into glucose, a simple sugar that travels through our bloodstream.

As glucose enters our bloodstream, the hormone insulin increases and acts as a gatekeeper to our cells, opening the cellular door to allow the glucose to enter and be used either for immediate energy or stored for later use—this combination of glucose and insulin results in quick energy delivery throughout our bodies. If there is extra glucose in our bloodstream, insulin helps our body store this excess glucose in our fat cells to be accessed later. When our bodies need energy and there is no food handy, it turns to these fat cells for energy.

As long as insulin levels are high, the stored energy is locked in fat cells. When insulin levels start to drop, the cells are unlocked, and we can start using the stored fat as energy. When we have increased levels of insulin due to consuming high carbs, more often than not, we prevent the body from switching to fat burning from glucose burning. This is where our natural metabolic flexibility breaks down.

When all the glucose in our bloodstream has been distributed and the energy from stored fat is not easily accessible due to the presence of insulin, we begin to feel sluggish, hungry, and start craving more food. So, we end up eating once again. And if the food we eat is high in carbohydrates, more insulin is released, restarting the cycle of energy consumption and storage all over again. When our body is constantly saturated with insulin, it takes a toll on us - we age faster and begin to develop insulin resistance, leading to metabolic disorders and weight gain. To stop this cycle and return to a state of burning stored fat, we need to activate the body's ability to access the extra fat we carry around, use it for energy, and improve our overall metabolic health. Fat has negligible insulin response and digests more slowly than carbohydrates, helping us feel fuller for longer. By limiting carbohydrate consumption, we allow insulin levels to fall, which enables metabolic flexibility, allowing our bodies to access fat stores to provide the energy required to function.

The fat-burning zone is the time when insulin is low, and our bodies use stored fat, not glucose, as energy. Reduced cravings for unhealthy foods, improved focus and concentration, more mental and physical energy, improved skin appearance, in addition to a healthy weight and body composition are some added advantages. So now that we know that our bodies are amazing and complex metabolic machines, we can be on our way to returning to a healthier and metabolically flexible state.

"The doctor of the future will no longer treat the human frame with drugs, but rather will cure and prevent disease with nutrition."
Thomas Edison

4

WHY ARE SUGARS BAD?

"Last generation we waged a war against tobacco. This generation we need to wage a war against sugar — for sugar is the new tobacco."

Glucose is a simple sugar molecule that is the primary fuel for our body. Unfortunately, glucose is usually combined with other forms of sugars; sucrose is half glucose and half fructose, most fruit sugars are primarily fructose, the sugar in milk is called lactose. Modern food processing has taken the sugars that have been bound together with chemical bonds in nature to make starch. Normally, during digestion, it takes a while to break these bonds in starches into glucose. But modern manufacturing has now been able to break these starch molecules into individual sugar molecules and still disguise them as starches. Simply put, a piece of bread has the equivalent of four teaspoons of sugar (four grams of sugar in each teaspoon) in it even though it doesn't taste sweet, which explains the high glycemic index of white bread. Likewise, there are 12 teaspoons of sugar in a can of soda.

Another belief is that natural sugar is healthy, but it is not so. Whether honey, jaggery or orange juice, they are all still sugars and can all spike your blood sugar levels. Juices are devoid of fiber and polyphenols and mainly contain fructose, one of the biggest drivers of obesity, fatty liver, and insulin resistance.

We have all been told time and again that sugar consumption is bad for our health. Yet, a majority of our calories come from both obvious and hidden sources of sugar in our diet. These hidden sugars are found in grains like rice, wheat, ragi, millet, and corn. As far as the perils of high sugars go, there is no ambiguity! We do not realize the importance of this until we develop some health issues. But who doesn't have a sweet tooth?!

Let us look at the complications and consequences of a high sugar diet. You will be surprised to know that most of the common illnesses are linked to sugars. The first thing to understand is that sugar has no nutritional value; it has 'empty' calories – no vitamins, minerals, essential fatty acids, or essential amino acids. Without these nutrients, you could land up with malnutrition and deficiencies, which prevents your body from performing its functions optimally. Sugars are also known to decrease the absorption of minerals and increase their excretion at the same time. Minerals like chromium, copper, zinc and magnesium are necessary to metabolize the calories we consume. While sugars don't provide any, they use the minerals stored in the body for their own metabolism, thereby depriving other important bodily functions of these nutrients.

Sugars also decrease the body's ability to resist infection because when blood glucose goes up, the activity of the white blood cells comes down. This makes it difficult to fight off pathogens, thus making us susceptible to infections. Eating any kind of sugar has the potential to reduce our body's defenses by 70 per cent for up to six hours, according to some researchers. If you go back in history, world war concentration camp survivors were found to be immune to infections. This was replicated in healthy volunteers who were put on a five-day fast, and with every fasting day, as blood sugars declined, the ability of white blood cells to kill bacteria increased. Vitamin C is not manufactured in humans but is concentrated in our white blood cells through a gradient. Glucose competes for the same pumps that pump vitamin C into our cells. Hence, higher the blood sugar, the more is the glucose in the cells, and lesser is the vitamin C. This translates to the reduced defensive ability of the white blood cells due to a deficiency of vitamin C.

Fig. 9: Sugar levels in common foods and what we actually consume

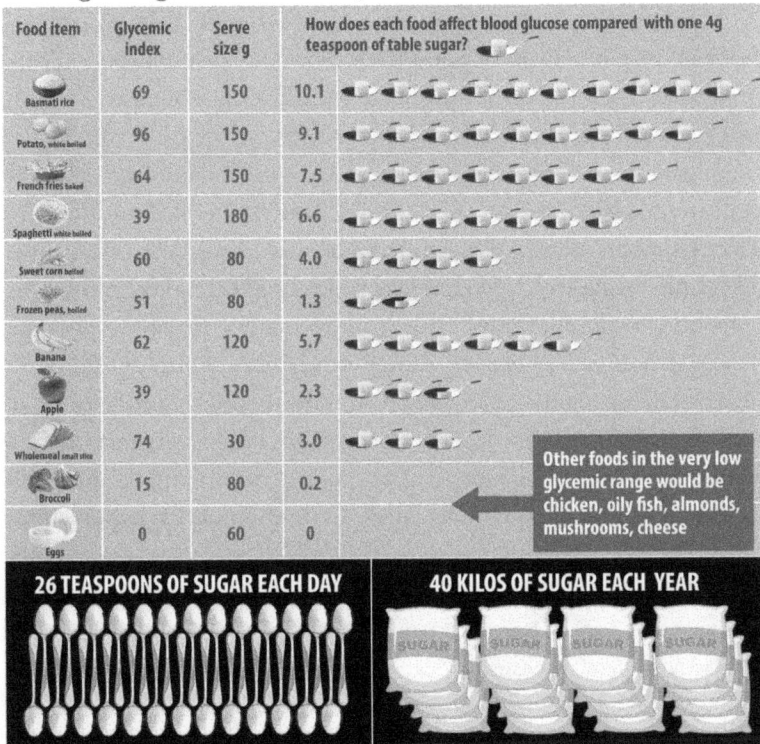

Food item	Glycemic index	Serve size g	How does each food affect blood glucose compared with one 4g teaspoon of table sugar?
Basmati rice	69	150	10.1
Potato, white boiled	96	150	9.1
French fries baked	64	150	7.5
Spaghetti white boiled	39	180	6.6
Sweet corn boiled	60	80	4.0
Frozen peas, boiled	51	80	1.3
Banana	62	120	5.7
Apple	39	120	2.3
Wholemeal small slice	74	30	3.0
Broccoli	15	80	0.2
Eggs	0	60	0

Other foods in the very low glycemic range would be chicken, oily fish, almonds, mushrooms, cheese

26 TEASPOONS OF SUGAR EACH DAY

40 KILOS OF SUGAR EACH YEAR

(Source: Dr. David Unwin)

The acceptable daily dose of added sugar is 6-8 tsp, but we consume close to 25-26 tsp every day. Inappropriate intake of sugars creates unstable blood glucose, which directly affects our higher mental functions. When blood sugars are low, it is called hypoglycemia, and when high, it is called hyperglycemia.

But, when we eat something like protein or fat or vegetables with fiber, the blood sugar remains stable. Alterations in the blood glucose levels give rise to irritability, lack of energy and lack of focus. More importantly, it leads to cravings as the brain sends out signals that the energy sources are depleting. Glucose also affects your moods as it can stimulate serotonin, a 'feel-good hormone,' and gives the 'sugar rush'.

Now coming to the dreaded cancer, the rapidly multiplying cells need a constant source of energy which comes from the breakdown of sugars. They thrive on glycolytic metabolism. Hence low sugars and high ketones can inhibit cancer growth.

Sugars can also cause dysregulation of hormones and neurotransmitters. Hormones are our body's chemical messengers. They travel in our bloodstream to tissues or organs and affect many different processes. Neurotransmitters affect our immediate behavior and emotions. Some important examples of this dysregulation are polycystic ovary syndrome, which is linked to menstrual irregularities and infertility. Dysregulation of neurotransmitters can lead to decreased libido, depression and anxiety in women. In men, it can cause gynecomastia and erectile dysfunction. In children, it can lead to attention deficit hyperactivity disorder.

High sugars are known to cause low-grade chronic inflammation, giving rise to several conditions like cardiovascular and cerebrovascular diseases. It can also cause premature ageing and Alzheimer's disease. Non-alcoholic fatty liver disease is increasing at an alarming rate, along with obesity, diabetes and abdominal weight gain. Though it was seen in older individuals, it is now common even in youngsters due to the popularity of infant formula food and carbonated drinks.

Several friendly microbes in our body modulate not only local but also systemic immunity. Disturbance in this population can upset our immune system and give rise to autoimmune diseases. Sugars selectively feed the pathogenic bacteria, which proliferate and start producing toxins. Unbalanced gut flora and toxins can lead to gastrointestinal symptoms. Other issues include hypothyroidism, pancreatic disease, and dental issues. Cavities are a result of bacteria that feed on sugar and create acid that destroys our teeth.

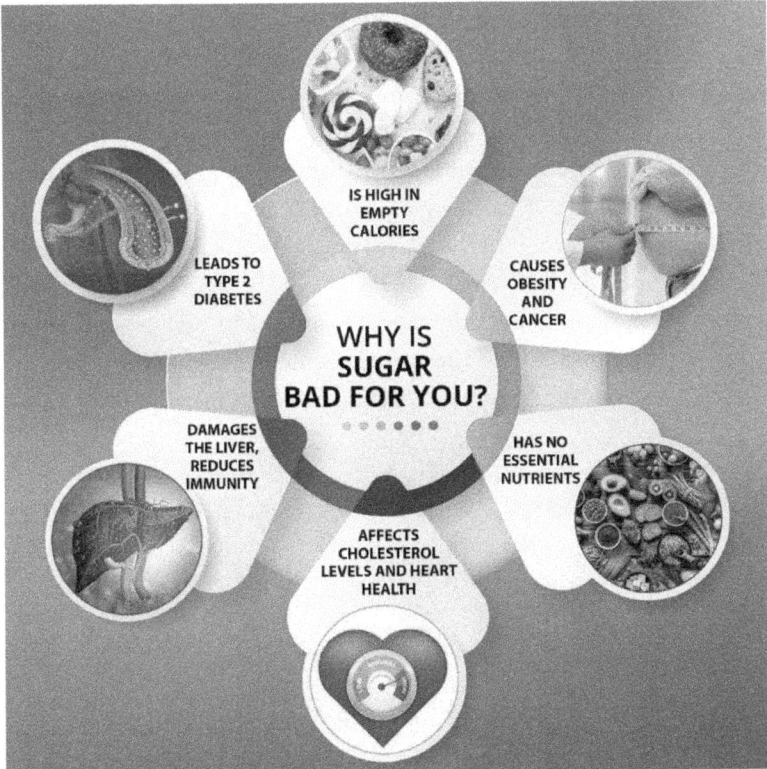

Fig. 10: Reasons to avoid sugars

Sugars promote insulin resistance in two ways, one of which is through fructose and non-alcoholic fatty liver disease. Another is through unstable blood sugars triggering constant high insulin, ultimately leading to insulin resistance that is linked to several degenerative conditions, obesity and high blood cholesterol. The body tends to convert excessive glucose into triglycerides as insulin promotes lipogenesis by taking excess sugar and converting it into fat.

Once the brain gets insulin resistant, it cannot access glucose. There is such a strong link between insulin resistance and dementia that they now even call it type-3 diabetes. Insulin resistance also promotes metabolic syndrome or syndrome X, which is a combination of all the above conditions.

Advanced glycation end-products or AGE are proteins that become glycated due to exposure to sugars. They are linked to degeneration and inflammation. They also damage collagen and elastin, which are essential to maintain the firmness and elasticity of the skin. Excessive sugar can damage these proteins leading to saggy skin and wrinkles. While ageing is inevitable, by reducing sugar intake, we can delay the changes. Sugars give rise to cravings, increase mood swings and make us eat more frequently. They are one of the most addictive substances like tobacco, alcohol and drugs. Now that you understand the mechanisms of the profound damage that sugars can cause, it is time to take remedial measures.

"If the current trend continues, for the first time in human history the younger generation will have a shorter lifespan than the current generation"

5

PROCESSED AND
REFINED FOODS

*'A poor woman who cooks her food at home has a better diet than
a rich woman who outsources her kitchen'*

It is indeed true that technological advancement and human development do not always go hand in hand. While technological advances are supposed to make human life easy and comfortable, is it really the case when it concerns our health? Today, most of us are addicted to processed food.

Owing to our busy lifestyle, eating something on the go is the norm. However, we must realize the harm these ready-to-eat, processed food items can do to our health. Scientists and food experts have learned that consuming processed foods can lead to obesity, type 2 diabetes, and many other chronic diseases. Processing is essentially the canning, frying, dehydrating, cooking, or freezing of food products and is done to increase a product's shelf-life. Where baked beans only last for one day in ordinary circumstances, canned beans can last for a year or two.

Processed and refined foods are deficient in nutrients but dense in calories; however, we find them tempting as they are delicious. The excessive concentration of additives such as sugar, sodium, taste enhancers and fats in processed food make it tasty. These foods are also chemically processed to improve their taste, texture, and expiry date.

A simple way to identify processed foods is to check the label. It is undoubtedly processed food if the label has a long list of unrecognizable and complicated names.

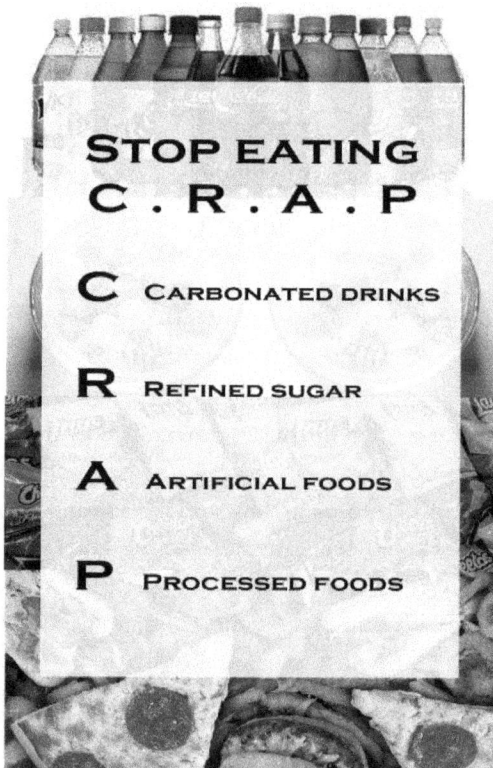

Fig. 11: Ultra-processed foods that can kill!

Many studies conclude that people who consume a great amount of ultra-processed foods tend to develop heart disease and die earlier than those who consume food in its original form. Heavily processed foods often have a high content of sugar, fat, and calories. Many of these foods can lead to an increased risk of health problems, such as obesity, high blood pressure, cancer, and depression, which can in turn lead to heart disease or premature death.

A person can substitute ultra-processed food with green leafy vegetables, healthy fats, nuts and seeds to balance the diet and make it healthier. The key is to create a healthy food choice. Every time you feel like snacking on a pack of chips, eat some nuts or seeds instead.

Additives are mostly used in processed meats for preservation, bacterial control, and to enhance the flavor and color. They are associated with a higher risk of stomach and esophagus cancer. According to an American Academy of Pediatrics publication, the use of artificial food colors may contribute to attention deficit hyperactivity disorder. Additives remove fiber, omega-3 fatty acids (anti-inflammatory), vitamins and minerals (micro-nutrients) from the food product. They also add more omega-6 fatty acids (pro-inflammatory), emulsifiers (which can erode intestinal mucous membranes), trans-fats, nitrates, and fructose to processed and refined foods. Additives in food lead to an increased risk of obesity, cardiovascular disease, liver diseases, and cancer in children and adults. It is imperative that we educate ourselves when it comes to eating. So, here is a comprehensive list of the most common processed food items that you need to watch out for.

- Frozen or ready-to-eat meals
- Baked goods like pizza, cakes, and pastries
- Breakfast cereal
- Desserts and ice-cream
- Chips and other packed snacks
- Instant noodles and soups

- Processed meat, such as sausages, salami, nuggets, fish fingers, and ham
- Beverages and other sugar-based drinks

Processed foods items:

- Are rich in fat, sugar, and salt
- Are low in fiber and micronutrients
- Have preservatives - chemicals that prevent the food from going bad
- Contain hydrogenated fats and additives

It is imperative that we know what goes into our meals or better still, that we make it ourselves. That way, we can measure and control the right amount of nutrients without the risk of unhealthy additives or empty calories.

Fig: 12: Results of healthy eating

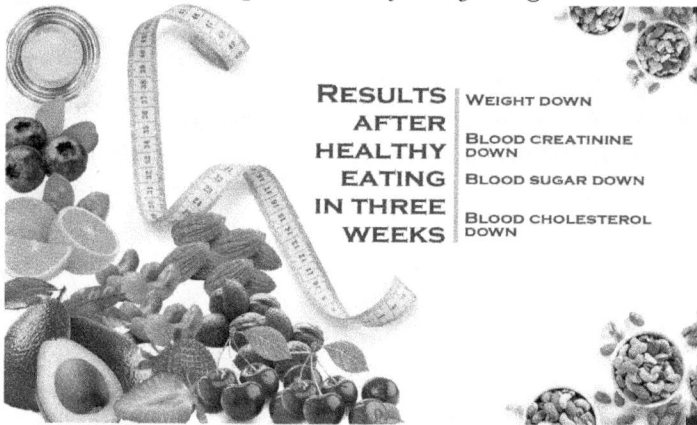

RESULTS AFTER HEALTHY EATING IN THREE WEEKS

WEIGHT DOWN

BLOOD CREATININE DOWN

BLOOD SUGAR DOWN

BLOOD CHOLESTEROL DOWN

"Came from a plant, eat it; was made in a plant, don't."
Michael Pollan

6

WHY VEGETABLE OILS ARE NOT WHAT THEY SEEM TO BE?

Whether we go back 100,000 years or 100 years, to our hunter gatherer ancestors or to our great grandparents, there is no historical precedent for widespread vegetable oil consumption.
-   Jeff Nobbs

From the 1960s, we were told that fats and oils are damaging for our health and can lead to conditions like cardiovascular diseases. As a society we have been conditioned to believe that unsaturated fats from vegetable and seed oils are better and that butter, ghee, and other saturated fats are unhealthy. In fact, the reverse is true. The type of fats we eat matters. Let us look at the history behind this misunderstanding.

The vegetable oil industry was born in the early 1900's. Those oils were first used during the industrial revolution to lubricate machinery. Then they figured out how to harden them, and bleach them to look white, and make them into soap.

When it started looking a lot like lard, they started to sell it as a food or vegetable oil. Those industries who were originally making soap using fatty acids, figured out how to make vegetable oils stable and fluid in bottles. They started to influence nutrition science in the 1940s with brilliant advertising campaigns. They then recommended that you start eating vegetable oils to prevent a heart attack with no real scientific evidence.

The Most Dangerous Cooking Oils That You Can Possibly Use

Though these cooking oils are called vegetable oils, none of them come from vegetables. They come from seeds and beans and there is not a single vegetable in any of these oils. So why are they called vegetable oils? It is a marketing gimmick because vegetable oil just sounds better and healthier than seed oil or bean oil. These oils just didn't exist before 1979 and you could barely find these seed oils in our food. But nowadays, you almost can't buy a food that doesn't have them. In the process, from 1979 to now, we have had an epidemic of obesity and autoimmune diseases, and all inflammatory conditions have gotten worse. Around ten years after these trans-fat hardened oils were marketed and sold to people, we started seeing an increase in morbidity and mortality due to heart diseases. Is it possible that seed oils might have something to do with it. This is because these seed oils are not natural. You cannot squeeze out the oil from soy beans like you can with an olive or like the oil you get from a coconut, or like the oil you get from meats, which naturally appear.

Why Should You Avoid Vegetable Oils?

Vegetable oils were 'invented' 120 plus years ago and we have increased our consumption of seed oil considerably in our country.

Any processed food (that is made in a factory) that you buy probably has this oil in it or some variety of it.

No oil is going to come out of a thousand kilo of seeds if you just squeeze them. Harsh chemicals and heat and all kinds of catalysts in a huge factory setting are needed to get the oil out of these seeds. And that is the part of what makes them so unnatural and so unhealthy.

If you visit a vegetable oil factory you will see what a brutal process it is to extract oil out of a bean or a seed. The product is an opaque and rancid fluid that is chemically extracted. If hexane is used as a solvent for extraction, the bad smelling grey liquid has to be deodorized. The oils that come from these seeds are unsaturated and that also is not natural. They have to harden the vegetable oil or make them solid through a process called hydrogenation. Even though they appear solid at room temperature like real saturated fats, they are not natural.

In a Minnesota coronary survey, people on vegetable oil or the so-called heart-healthy diet died at much higher rates from cancer. But nobody could figure out why that was happening, and since they believed that vegetable oils would help people prevent heart disease, they probably ignored the cancer effect. When you look at the data, it is confusing.

Large observational processes show that there is a risk from saturated fats and a benefit from omega-3 and omega-6 oils. Then there is other data from randomized trials that show the opposite. When you have people eat only vegetable oil, they do worse. Most bakery products and processed foods are made from these dangerous vegetable oils – because they are inexpensive and thought to be "heart healthy".

If you want to restore your health, you need to see how many processes your food goes through from the source till it reaches your plate. If it is more than one or two, it is probably not good or healthy for you.

When compared to these chemically processed oils, which we are told is healthy, churning butter is a simpler process that can be done at home. So don't outsource your cooking – home-made or home cooked food is the best!

Hydrogenated unsaturated fat is unhealthy and increases the risk of inflammatory diseases. Unsaturated fats are highly unstable and dangerous in the oil form. The huge worry about vegetable oils is that when they are heated and exposed to light (even if they are left out in a bottle), they will oxidize and degrade, or go rancid.

When you put them under heat, they break down into degraded oxidation products, some of which are known toxins. Oxidation causes inflammation in your body and most of us take antioxidants to prevent that.

Oxidized LDL is what is thought to provoke that unstable plaque that causes heart blockage. When you feed your body hydrogenated unsaturated fats instead of saturated fats, your cell membranes are being made up of these inferior fats. This is again going to increase the risk of oxidative damage.

Indians are eating frightening amounts of refined vegetable oils, seed oils and omega-6 fats, all of which contribute to inflammation and chronic diseases. So, if all of our cell membranes are built up of these inferior fats since the last 30-40 years, it is no wonder that we all have oxidative damage. Because of these oils, we are more afflicted with autoimmune conditions, we are aging quicker, and we are falling apart quicker.

The most dangerous vegetable oil is canola oil and is derived from rapeseeds. There are other oils like cottonseed oil, safflower oil and soybean oil. Basically, any unsaturated oil that is hydrogenated is a definite no-no. So, if you are using any of these vegetable oils, please replace them with the good saturated fats. Processed food is so much cheaper and easier and tastier to eat. Please remember that all fast food has unsaturated hydrogenated oils in them. They all use the seed oils but call it vegetable oils or even say organic vegetable oils for marketing reasons, but there's no such thing. You may have saved time and money by buying the processed food with the unsaturated fats, but you're going to end up paying the ultimate price with poor health, suffering disease and death.

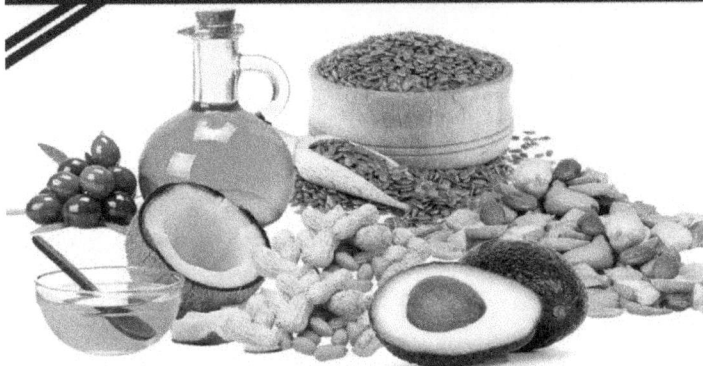

Fig. 13: Healthy oils that are safe to use

Every cell membrane in your body is made up of fat and cholesterol. You should be using saturated real fats and real oils that are extracted from animals or plants without chemicals, without heat, and without chemical catalysts. The saturated oils you want to be cooking with are: Oils from grass-fed animal and vegetable oils like avocado oil, organic extra virgin olive oil, and coconut oil. Cold-pressed oils like flaxseed oil, walnut oil and hemp seed oil are great for topping a wide variety of dishes. Organic extra virgin olive oil is also great for cooking at very low heat. You can also use ghee and butter in your cooking. Mayonnaise that is made from avocado oil or olive oil is a good alternative. Vegetable and seed oils are the types of oils used in most restaurants, especially for frying, and they can even be used in seemingly healthy salad dressings. When eating out, please do ask what kinds of oils the kitchen uses and request for a healthier alternative for a healthier life.

"Processed oils have been pushed past their heat tolerance and have become rancid in the processing." – Lisa Howard, author of The Big Book of Healthy Cooking Oils

7

LIFESTYLE DISEASES

"Genetics only load the gun, but it is the environment that pulls the trigger."
— *Francis Collins*

A 2016 study revealed that the death rate due to lifestyle diseases had escalated from 37.09% in 1990 to 61.8% in 2016. Another 2017 study showed that non-communicable diseases (NCDs) depended entirely on lifestyle practices and could kill around 40 million people each year. Reports released by the Centre for Science and Environment (CSE) has also confirmed that 61% of all deaths in India are due to lifestyle diseases.

The situation is so bad that even school children are being diagnosed with lifestyle disorders in recent times. Spending unending hours on digital devices with no physical or outdoor activity can be one of the main reasons. Although work from home and online classes are unavoidable, we must learn to make some changes for our better health. With limited or no physical activity, we tend to become lethargic or sick. Additionally, kids have unlimited access to junk food like pizzas, burgers, fries, and carbonated drinks these days.

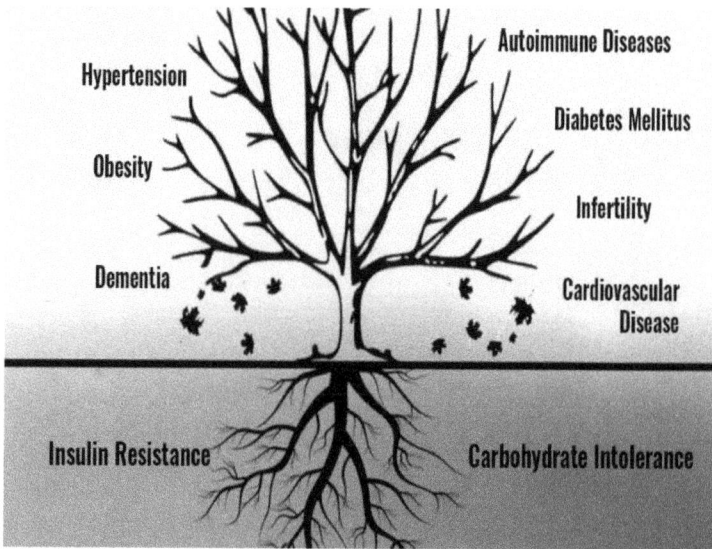

Fig. 14: Interplay between insulin resistance and lifestyle diseases

Studies have revealed that around 15 million people between the ages of 30-50 die prematurely every year from cardiovascular diseases, cancer, diabetes, and high blood pressure. Four decades ago, a 30-year-old son admitting their 60-year-old parents to the hospital with ailments was the norm. Sadly, today, we see 60-year-old parents hospitalizing their 30-year-old son for the same reasons and even losing them at a tender age. Making a few changes in your daily food routine goes a long way. Once you make these dietary changes, you will be able to get your health back on track.

I am writing this book to tell you that nothing is irreversible. The fact that a cut on your hand heals by itself proves that the human body is built in such a way that it can heal and get back to its original state—provided you give it a chance. So, never underestimate the power of your body. Many blame their genes for their diseases. Well, genes only have a 10-20% role to play here. Genes are like seeds. They can only sprout according to the provided environment— diseases manifest only if the environment is optimal.

Let me explain this with a simple story: Two identical twins lived in the countryside. After their schooling, they parted ways to pursue different careers; while one stayed back in the village and took to agriculture, the other chose a posh city life. The twins met again after 20 long years and were dumbfounded on seeing each other. The man who stayed back in the village looked young and fit while the other looked obese and unhealthy. The one who went to the city adopted the fast-food and party culture, whereas the one who stayed back continued to toil in the field, ate healthy food and remained youthful and energetic. Though they had identical genes, they ended up looking different because they grew up in different environments and cultures.

Another worrying trend is the increase in the incidence of cancer, an illness where abnormal cells divide quickly and uncontrollably to form tumors and destroy healthy body tissue. These cells also spread to other parts of the body, making it a deadly disease.

According to the World Cancer Report, based on the estimated cancer burden in India, there are about 1.16 million new cancer cases as of early 2020.

WHO studies have predicted that one in 15 Indians will die of cancer. These numbers are alarming. Most of us are exposed to cancer-causing elements every day. Excessive exposure to sunlight, passive smoking, and X-rays are few such.

We are all vulnerable. If you think about it, most of us would have been exposed to these risks at some point in our lives, but not all develop cancer.

Many people have cancer-related genes, but still do not suffer from the disease. This is because each person reacts differently to different carcinogenic substances and some people may have a stronger immune system that can fight cancer-causing cells. Dietary changes can also help fight the dreaded disease.

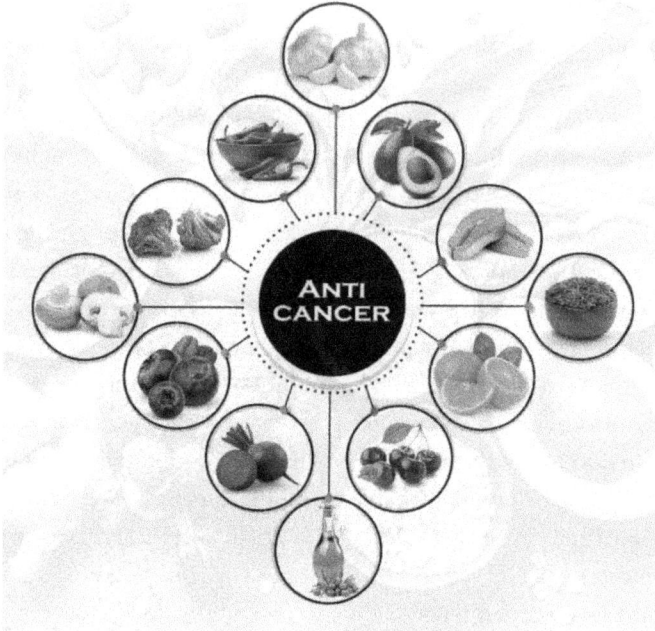

Fig. 15: Common foods protective against cancer

Even during the recent pandemic, there was much evidence that diabetes, hypertension and cardiovascular diseases contributed significantly to the adverse outcomes of coronavirus disease 2019 (COVID-19). Morbidly obese people were more likely to contract COVID-19 and also suffered from more severe complications with an increased requirement for mechanical ventilation. Those suffering with these lifestyle diseases are predisposed to more severe respiratory manifestations and infections due to chronic systemic inflammation and reduced immunity.

The LCHF diet can be extremely effective in reducing body weight and reducing systemic inflammation and may be considered as an adjuvant therapy for patients with respiratory compromise in the setting of these chronic diseases. To save yourself from lifestyle disorders, quit the 'bad' habits, keep a check on your weight and body mass index, get enough exercise every day and most importantly, eat right. Dietary habits and lifestyle choices play an important role, especially with regards to developing a robust immune system.

"To kill an error is as good a service as, and sometimes even better than, the establishing of a new truth or fact."
— Charles Darwin

8

OBESITY AND YOUR DIET

"Obesity is a problem that nearly every nation in the world is facing, but there is much that we can do to fix it."
- Richard Attias

Decimus Junius Juvenalis, the Roman poet, widely known as Juvenal, once said, "a healthy mind is in a healthy body". Buddha has also spoken on similar lines, "To keep the body in good health is a duty. Otherwise, we shall not be able to keep our mind strong and clear."

In today's world, it is easy to lose our balance and give in to the desires of our heart impulsively. In the rush of our day-to-day lives, there is significantly less time for self-care. After a long day at work, it is tempting to order-in from your favorite restaurant, and binge watch your favorite show. You may want to lie in bed as long as you can because, of course, there is a long, tiresome day awaiting you again. All this is acceptable if it was only for a day, but we are at risk of this becoming a routine, and in such cases, the dangers that can come with it are inevitable.

Obesity can be defined as excessive fat accumulation that poses a major health risk to an individual. The quantity of accumulated fat is assessed with the body mass index (BMI), which is a measure that considers the height and weight of the individual. If the BMI is above 30, it indicates that the individual is obese. If it is between 25 and 30, it suggests that the individual is overweight. Waist circumference, which denotes the fat distribution around the waist, is another important measure of obesity. Being overweight or obese has a negative impact on an individual. The chances of acquiring cancer, cardiovascular diseases, type 2 diabetes, osteoarthritis, infertility, irregular periods, non-alcoholic fatty liver, and obstructive sleep apnea are high in obese people. Another significant effect of obesity is that it affects the quality of life and often leads to psychological conditions such as depression, low self-esteem, shame, and guilt.

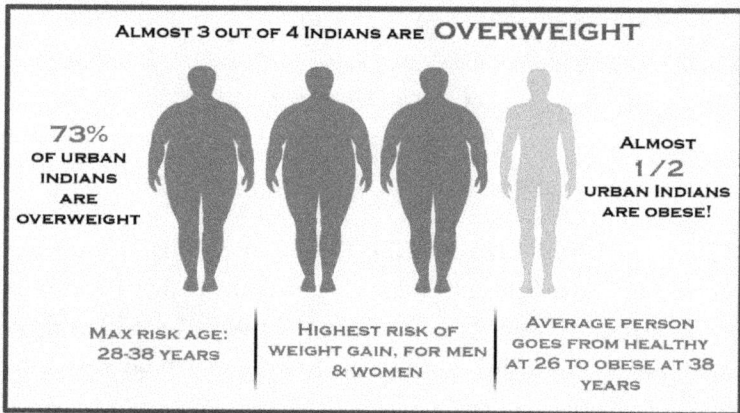

ALMOST 3 OUT OF 4 INDIANS ARE OVERWEIGHT

73% OF URBAN INDIANS ARE OVERWEIGHT

ALMOST 1/2 URBAN INDIANS ARE OBESE!

MAX RISK AGE: 28-38 YEARS

HIGHEST RISK OF WEIGHT GAIN, FOR MEN & WOMEN

AVERAGE PERSON GOES FROM HEALTHY AT 26 TO OBESE AT 38 YEARS

Fig 16: The 'large' problem at hand in our country.

One of the challenging questions about obesity is pinpointing what triggers the accumulation of fat, which ultimately results in obesity. One obvious cause is consuming much more calories than an individual requires for physiological processes of the body. Unhealthy eating habits, poor dietary habits, consumption of oily, starchy, and sweet food materials, and lack of sleep lead to hormonal changes and increased appetite.

Genetic factors, the basal metabolic rate, intake of medications like steroids and anti-depressants, hormonal contraception, hypothyroidism and polycystic ovarian syndrome [PCOS] are some other causes of obesity. On the other hand, several medical conditions are a result of obesity itself. It increases the risk of calcium and fat accumulation in blood vessels resulting in higher blood pressure and a higher level of triglycerides, leading to heart diseases and strokes. Consequent to very high carbohydrates consumed, the excess glucose gets accumulated in the bloodstream and liver, increasing the risk of diabetes, perceived to be a lifelong and chronic condition. If unnoticed or untreated, it can affect the heart, blood vessels, kidneys, nerves, skin, eyes, and brain.

Obesity has a significant role in triggering the growth of cancerous cells, with high chances of the uterus, cervix, ovaries, kidney, and prostate being affected. Inflammation of the visceral fat that covers these vital organs is a possible factor that triggers the growth of cancerous cells. Gastroesophageal reflux disease is a common condition in obese individuals, resulting in heartburn.

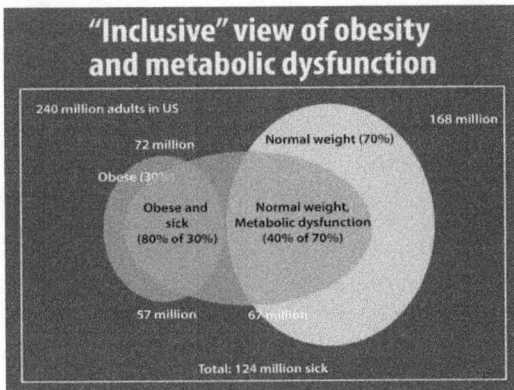

Fig 17: Inclusive View of Obesity and metabolic dysfunction
Polycystic ovarian syndrome, infertility issues, irregular menstrual

cycles and erectile dysfunction are other conditions that result from obesity. Sleep apnea is a disorder commonly affecting obese individuals, leading to a feeling of exhaustion despite a full night's sleep. Obesity is also one of the primary conditions that precipitates osteoarthritis. Stress exerted on weight-bearing joints and inflammation causes the cartilage to wear off.

Obesity and metabolic dysfunction

Obesity is primarily a hormonal disorder and the hormone involved is insulin as it is a fat-storing hormone. As the insulin level goes up, which happens in early diabetes and prediabetics, the fat tends to deposit around the waist, commonly known as belly fat. Insulin not only stores fat, but also locks it up. The most common cause for fatty liver was assumed to be over-consumption of alcohol thus far. Now there is evidence that excessive intake of sugar and carbs can give rise to non-alcoholic fatty liver. The best and the easiest way to reduce weight is to reduce the level of insulin in the blood or to reduce insulin resistance. The only way to do that is to avoid sugars and refined or processed carbohydrates because they spike insulin the most.

The rise of childhood obesity has placed the health of an entire generation at risk.
-Tom Vilsack

9

THE SECRET TO WEIGHT LOSS
LIES IN WHAT YOU EAT

"I eat everything I want. I have just changed what I want."
– Dr. Lucy Burns

If you are ready to lose weight and that belly fat, this chapter will bring it all together for you. Why do we gain fat in the first place? Is it because we are eating too many calories? Is it because we eat too often? Is it because we eat the wrong things? It is because of all these and more. Our ancestors, who had a strong genetic makeup, remained healthy for thousands of centuries and were successful in maintaining their weight. But now, the food we eat is not natural anymore and is causing a hormonal imbalance. While every other animal on the planet eats food from nature that is appropriate for their species, humans don't do that anymore.

The first issue is that we eat too often. Every other species on the planet does not necessarily have three square meals a day and snack every two hours. Likewise, our ancestors probably ate once or twice a day when they were hungry or were lucky enough to find food. And if they were not so lucky, they might even have gone without food for 2-3 days. So, there was a fasting pattern or a cycle built into their metabolism. Nowadays, access to food is easy and quick, thereby bypassing the fasting phase altogether.

Eating until satiety is the norm and definitely not several times a day. When we eat too often, we get stuck in the "eat and store" cycle. The average person has about 100 milligrams of glucose per deciliter and a total of 5 grams of glucose in 5 liters of blood. The body really likes to keep it in a tight range - when you are fasting, you might be at 80 to 85 milligrams, and after a meal it might be 120. If you eat whole food with protein like meat, and good fats, and non-starchy vegetables, these changes fluctuate slowly. In a diabetic or someone with insulin resistance, the blood sugar shoots up more rapidly. This amount of blood glucose is very toxic to the brain. It damages blood vessels, causing micro-vessel disease, which is the cause for kidney failure and blindness. It also causes neuropathy and is the leading cause of amputations.

Many times, people say that carbohydrate is the preferential fuel because the body uses it first. Well, it is not that the body prefers it - but that it has to use carbs first. And if you ate a hundred grams of carbohydrate, all of that glucose has to get into the bloodstream before it gets into the cells. This has to happen in a relatively short time period (before your next meal). Whatever extra carbohydrates you can't use before the next meal (the excess) has to be stored.

There are two types of energy that the body can store - carbohydrate and fat. We have a very limited or poor ability to store carbohydrates. Your muscles can hold about 1600 calories, and your liver can store about 400 calories. Why do we store energy? It's for survival. We need energy for movement, to generate heat and to think, to move, and to receive signals from the brain to control movement and metabolism.

However, fat is a much more efficient form of storage, and we can store 90 times the amount of carbohydrates, which is 180000 calories. This would keep us alive for three months.

The body can store excess energy as fat but it's the surplus glucose that most readily gets stored and converted into fat. If you want to lose weight or lose some fat, you have to understand that you can't burn fat if you keep adding carbs. If you put more carbs into your body before you burn the previous ones, you can't get to the fat-burning mode and can never lose that fat. In the presence of high insulin (which again is a result of those carbs), you can't burn fat. In the presence of high insulin, your body is busy making fat. Your body cannot make fat and burn fat at the same time.

Now, while we do want to reduce overall carbs, not all carbs are equally bad. Take bread for example - 70% of the weight in a slice of bread is net carbs (pure starch) and that starch is going to get converted into glucose. If we couple that with some jam, some orange juice, and some sugar in the coffee, it easily goes up to 100 grams of carbs in one meal. Now, let's look at a non-starchy vegetable like cabbage - 3% percent of its weight is carbs, which is absorbed much slower. Therefore, you will not load up on carbs by eating non-starchy vegetables. The two important factors here are quantity and speed - how much you eat and how quickly it gets converted to glucose in your body.

The cell is the metabolic machinery that's actually going to use glucose for energy. Glucose cannot become energy until it's in the cell and that is what insulin does. It unlocks the cell to allow the glucose through. The cell uses some of the glucose for energy and turns the rest of it into fat. If glucose stays within the normal range, the insulin required is very moderate. But if we have huge spikes of glucose, we need a ton of insulin to get that glucose into the cells. If we eat every four hours, that insulin doesn't even have time to come down to baseline before we load up on more carbs. While carbs drive high insulin, the frequency of eating amplifies it and the body has to make more and more insulin because the cells don't respond. This is when we develop insulin resistance.

A fat cell can expand more than any other cell in the body. In its shrunken state, it is about 10 microns or 10 micrometers, but it can grow 8,000 times. When we start pushing the limit of that capacity, it becomes inflamed. When we overload the fat cell, it starts leaking and is not a healthy fat cell anymore. This is when we develop the metabolic problems of insulin resistance such as metabolic syndrome, type-2 diabetes, cardiovascular disease, stroke, dementia, and so on.

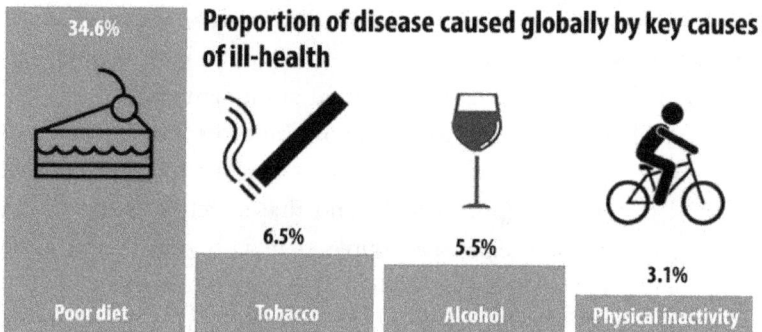

Fig. 18: Key causes of ill-health
(Source: Prof Simon Capewell, Professor of Clinical Epidemiology, University of Liverpool, analysis of Lancet global burden of disease report.)

An Unhealthy Diet Is the Highest Contributor to Ill-Health

If we go back several centuries ago, 100% of what we ate was from nature, unprocessed and unmodified. We ate meat, vegetables, nuts, and tubers - anything that we could hunt, capture, dig up, or pick. Around 8,000 years ago, we started agriculture but everything was still unprocessed and most of what we ate was still whole food. Around this time, humans had started using some naturals oils like olive oil. However, in the last 50 years, we have turned everything completely upside down. We eat white flour, sugar, plant oils processed with harsh chemicals and high heat; we eat food with preservatives, chemicals, artificial flavors, artificial sugars, and artificial colors. We have to realize that we come from a genetic background that needs natural, unprocessed and unmodified food, but we are not getting these anymore.

Processed foods are particularly bad because a lot of sugar is added to them to make food taste very good at a very, very low cost. So, avoiding these sugars is critical for weight loss. That includes white sugar, jaggery, and things with fructose like fruit juice concentrates. Another item to avoid is refined grains, white rice or polished rice, and instant oatmeal. Unrefined carbohydrates which are starchy are found in roots that grow underground like potatoes, tapioca, and yam, because these plants store carbohydrates for later use. The rise in glucose from these carbohydrates depends on how you make them, how much you eat, and how often.

Fruits are very controversial because they are natural food. Most fruits have a lot of fructose and fruit juices are worse because all of the fiber and pulp have been removed. Berries such as strawberries, raspberries, and blackberries are much better than other sweet fruits. Another thing to keep in mind is that many of the fruits that we eat today are different from the fruits that we ate 30-40 years ago. They are much sweeter as they have been genetically altered.

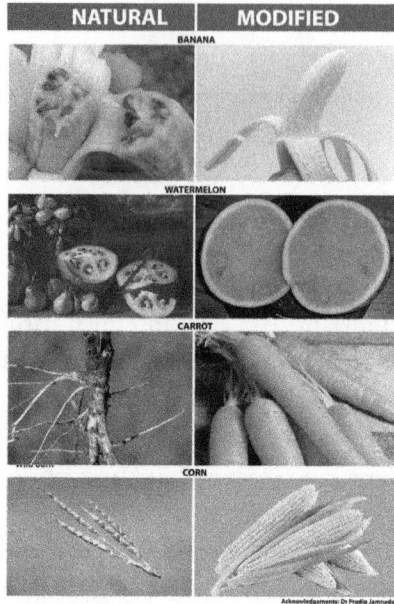

Fig. 19: Genetically modified fruits and vegetables

The bulk of the carbohydrates in your diet should be unrefined, non-starchy and more fibrous. This includes vegetables that grow above the ground. Because of the high fiber in them, they add bulk and give a sense of satiety. They are absorbed slowly, resulting in a very slow rise in blood glucose and insulin. Legumes and lentils are examples of carbohydrates that do not have much of an effect on insulin. They are very good vegetable sources of protein and can sometimes be combined with natural fats. Other non-root vegetables such as asparagus, peppers, broccoli, cauliflower, Brussel sprouts, eggplants, and leafy greens are carbohydrates which are safe and nutritious to consume. Remember to avoid refined and starchy carbohydrates, root vegetables, as well as fruit. Unrefined non-starchy carbohydrates such as legumes, lentils, and leafy green vegetables can be consumed in reasonable quantities.

"When diet is wrong, medicine is of no use.
When diet is correct, medicine is of no need."
Ayurvedic proverb

10

DIABETES AND YOUR DIET

I have high blood sugars, and Type 2 diabetes is not going to kill me.
But I just have to eat right, and exercise, and lose weight,
and watch what I eat, and I will be fine for the rest of my life."
-Tom Hanks.

Diabetes is on the rise in India, with at least two out of five adults being diabetic. No wonder India ranks second among the top 10 diabetic countries in the world. According to a study in *The Lancet*, the number of people with diabetes has risen from 108 million in 1998 to 422 million in 2014. The global prevalence of diabetes among adults over the age of 18 has increased to 8.5% as of 2014. Initially, diabetes was referred to as a rich man's disease. However, that isn't the case anymore. Studies have shown that diabetes is rapidly increasing among the middle and low-income groups of the society as well. Presumably, the number of people living with diabetes will rise to 642 million around the world by 2040.

Diabetes is a condition that occurs when your body does not properly produce or use the hormone insulin. When this insulin imbalance occurs, there is an increase in the blood sugar level. It is classified into two main types:

a) Type 1 diabetes

b) Type 2 diabetes

Type 1 diabetes occurs when there is no insulin production in the body. It is also referred to as juvenile diabetes and it is primarily detected in children and young adults. Type 2 diabetes occurs when the body produces inadequate insulin or does not function adequately. Apart from these two types of diabetes, there is pre-diabetes, which is a condition wherein the blood sugar levels are higher than expected but not high enough to warrant medication.

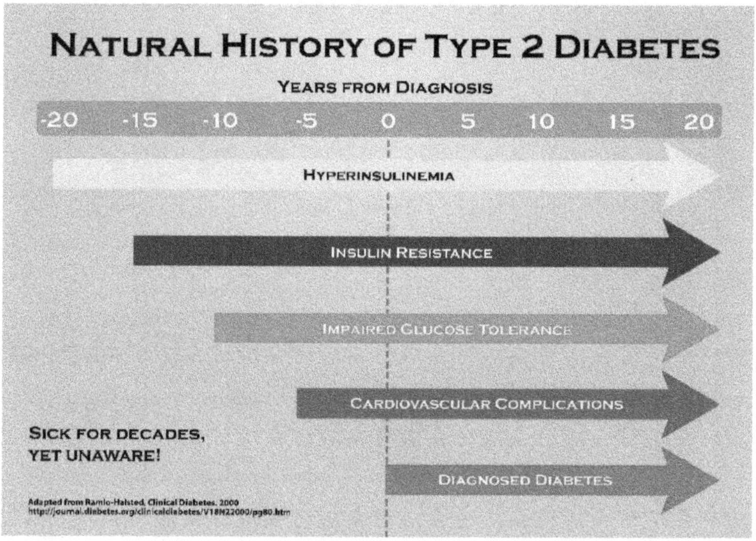

Fig. 20: Natural history of Type 2 Diabetes

How does diabetes develop?

If you are prediabetic with higher-than-normal blood sugar levels and do not make lifestyle modifications, you are at a risk of developing type 2 diabetes. Family history and genetics appear to play an important role, but the exact cause of prediabetes is unknown.

Lack of regular physical activity and being overweight seem to be important contributory factors. While prediabetes doesn't usually have any symptoms, increased thirst, frequent urination, excessive hunger or fatigue can indicate that you may have developed diabetes. Both adults and children with prediabetes are prone to developing type 2 diabetes.

Even as a prediabetic, damage of your heart, blood vessels and kidneys may have started. But the progression from prediabetes to type 2 diabetes can be stopped if you take precautionary steps. Eating healthy foods, ensuring daily physical activity and controlling your weight can help bring your blood sugar level back to normal.

Hard Hitting Facts about Diabetes:

1. **People with diabetes:** Diabetes affects around 70 million people in India. That's a very significant percentage of our population with full-blown type 2 diabetes. Out of those people, 50% do not even know that they have it. So as high as the numbers are, these problems are still under-diagnosed.

2. **Diabetes can lead to other health problems:** It is the number one reason for amputations, be it toes, or feet, or fingers, and so forth. It is the leading cause of blindness and can result in kidney failure and a requirement for dialysis.

3. **Diabetes can lead to death:** It is the number seven overall cause of death.

4. **Diabetes leads to metabolic syndrome:** Diabetes is the primary causative mechanism for metabolic syndrome or syndrome-X which essentially is associated with higher blood pressure, increased cardiovascular disease, and increased risk for stroke.

5. **Blood sugar is not the only problem:** We need to understand that out of the two factors - the blood glucose and the insulin - the insulin is the real problem. So how can we address it? We need to reduce the insulin by not eating those foods that most trigger insulin. We need to give the body a chance to burn off some of that fuel before we put more in.

6. **90% of diabetes is reversible:** Though there will always be a few cases that are just too far gone, the vast majority of cases can be reversed. It is overloading of primarily sugar and carbohydrates that triggers insulin. If you stop adding so much of it, and so often, the body will have a chance to burn something off. If you keep eating sugar and carbs, you are going to just perpetuate the condition and make it worse.

"Before diagnosis of Type 2 diabetes, there is a long silent scream from the liver." – Professor Roy Taylor

11

INSULIN RESISTANCE

The food we eat is either the culprit or the cure
– Dr. Benjamin Bickman

Traditionally diabetes has been viewed to be a chronic, progressive and irreversible disease and presumed to require medications lifelong. The similar is true for hypertension. We assume that people are incapable or unwilling to do the necessary changes to reverse the condition. The human body is programed to work in a balanced manner. If we upset that balance, diseases and illnesses manifest. To restore back normalcy, certain steps and measures need to be taken. Rather than treating the disease itself, we need to try to address the factors that lead to it. Insulin resistance is one such deterrent in the management of diabetes. The term insulin resistance implies that the body is resisting the actions of the hormone insulin resulting in increased blood sugar. Why does it occur? Constant high blood sugars make the cells in our body resistant to the regulatory action of insulin.

When we eat food, it is broken down into carbohydrates, fats, proteins and micronutrients and absorbed into the bloodstream. Carbohydrates raise the blood sugar the most, and hence generate the strongest insulin response. Proteins lead to a moderate insulin response and fats, a negligible one.

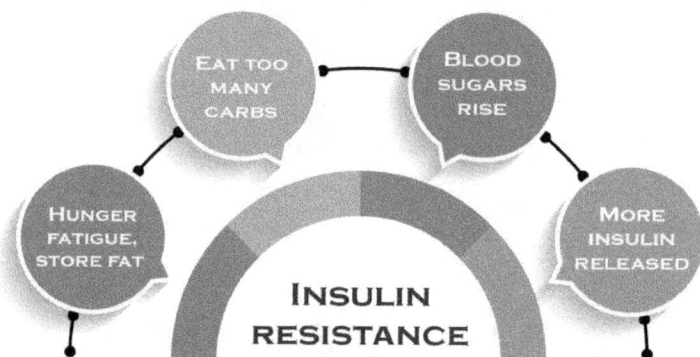

Fig. 21: Vicious cycle of insulin resistance.

The total amount of sugar in our blood is just 5 grams or one tea spoon. The carbohydrates we consume contribute to the rise in blood sugars. Even though our blood volume is high, there is a concentration beyond which the sugars need to be transported into the cells. Once the glucose in these cells required for the body's functioning are expended, the rest is converted to glycogen and fat, which is deposited in the surrounding tissue and liver. Hence, cells can hold much more 'calories' than blood! But once the cell reserves are full, the sugar overloads the blood stream. Basically, the cells start resisting the insulin action and it leads to increasing blood sugars. Unfortunately, conventional treatment is aimed at lowering the blood sugars by using different drugs to make the 'compromised' cells more insulin sensitive.

Eventually, the demand for insulin is so much that the pancreas can't keep up, thereby requiring insulin injections. So, treatment just helps lower the blood sugar, without addressing the root cause be it excessive carbs or the consequences of damage at a cellular level such as abdominal obesity, cardiovascular disease, or raised lipids, all part of the 'metabolic syndrome'. Rather than forcing the excess blood sugar into the cells, we should limit the intake of carbs that get converted into blood sugar.

Insulin resistance is hardly addressed as we are not focusing on the source of the problem which is making diabetes a chronic or lifelong condition. While exercise can help reduce insulin resistance, it has no effect on reversing the adverse effects of chronic damage to the system. Likewise, increased weight is a consequence of high carbs and weight loss is not a solution if the input remains constant or increases. Nutritionists advise that a majority of your calories must be from carbs and they also recommend 1-2 portions of fruits per day. Whether it is fresh or frozen, canned or juiced, or even dried, fruits in general contribute to higher sugar intake, even if it is a natural and unprocessed source. If you are not insulin resistant, you can still eat some fresh fruit. But if you have insulin resistance and you eat a large portion of fruits, it will surely cause a further imbalance.

Consumption of non-fat dairy with only protein and sugar is a fad these days. Whole fat dairy, on the other hand, would slow down the sugar absorption. Nonetheless, dairy still has enough sugar to spike the blood sugar. Even though you have not consumed any chocolate or ice cream, you have still consumed a lot of sugar. It is therefore a problem of over-consumption, and not just the high blood sugar.

When we overload on carbs, we trigger insulin to increase the fat reserves. If we do the opposite of the above by decreasing the intake of carbs, the cells would start burning off all the stored fat. If we take steps to prevent the insulin trigger, it would prevent cellular overloading. A few things we need to do to stop triggering insulin is to cut out sugars, reduce carbs, and eat fewer meals. This gives the cells a window to overcome the overloading and to start burning up some of those fat reserves.

To curb your snacking urge, have moderate proteins and eat more healthy fats. The longer you go without eating between meals, the more time you give those cells a chance to start using up some of that stored fat. By increasing the demand for energy, exercising helps to burn some of the stored fat and also increases the insulin sensitivity of the muscles. Stress is another factor that pushes the body to raise blood sugars to give us enough fuel to handle the situation. When the blood sugar goes up, so does the insulin. Hence, stress and cortisol actually increase insulin resistance.

Meditation, yoga, breathing exercises and listening to calm music can contribute towards managing your sugars better. Exercising all day long and starving may seem to work for a while, but it is difficult to sustain and the success is temporary. It is also a myth that weight management is paramount as thin people can also suffer from diabetes and its complications. It is more important to determine what it takes to be healthy! And remember insulin resistance is reversible as long as we take these remedial steps:

1. Low carb diet
2. Intermittent fasting
3. Exercise
4. Less stress
5. Adequate sleep

Hard hitting facts about insulin resistance:

1. **People with insulin resistance:** Over 150 million Indians have insulin resistance and out of all those people, 90% don't even know they have it. The people who have it don't know why they have it, so they are not attempting to make any changes.

   Insulin resistance is also called pre-diabetes or pre-type 2 diabetes because very often, or even typically, insulin resistance can progress to type-2 diabetes within 5-10 years. So, we need to understand that these are progressive mechanisms that wear out the body.

2. **People who are overweight:** To get a true idea of how big this problem is, we must understand that the number one cause of weight gain is insulin resistance. A majority of people in India are overweight. However, neither do all obese persons have high insulin resistance and nor do all thin people have low insulin resistance, but there is a pretty close correlation between obesity and insulin resistance.

3. **Continuum of insulin resistance:** When we talk about insulin resistance and diabetes, we need to understand that it is a continuum - insulin resistance and diabetes are not two different things. They are just different degrees of the same thing. So, you go all the way from insulin sensitive to mildly insulin resistant, to moderate, to severely insulin resistant, and to full-blown diabetes. When you have broken the system, high levels of insulin still cannot get the blood sugar down. So how do you reverse diabetes and insulin resistance? You have to eat less sugar, less carbs, and eat fewer meals. You need to get some exercise and work on reducing your stress. All these things are the factors that drive insulin and insulin resistance. By reducing them, you will give the body a chance to recover.

Insulin resistance in the muscles causes diabetes
Insulin resistance in the brain causes dementia
Insulin resistance in the eyes causes blindness
Insulin resistance in the liver causes fatty liver
Insulin resistance in the kidneys causes kidney failure

12

IS THERE A CURE FOR DIABETES?

Fight the staggering rise of type-2 diabetes
by simply learning to cook healthy fresh food -
it's fun, and it could save your life!
Jamie Oliver

A lot of people are normalizing their blood sugars through lifestyle changes and medications – but is there a permanent cure for diabetes? The general impression is that diabetes is a chronic, and incurable disease. With modern research and advances in treatments, one can hope for a cure for diabetes. In type-1 disease there is a complete lack of insulin and in type-2 diabetes there is insulin resistance or too much insulin. So, they are really two opposites but we will only be discussing type-2 diabetes. Cure is to relieve a person of the symptoms of a disease, and to heal or restore good health.

Simply looking for a way to relieve the symptoms of a disease does not suffice. The absence of symptoms does not mean that we are healthy. One needs to first understand how and why the disease occurs. Illnesses develop as a result of a long-term imbalance. Cure or treatment denotes medicine or medication used to treat the symptoms, but not necessarily to reverse a disease. While there may be a pill to treat a symptom, it will not change the underlying condition itself.

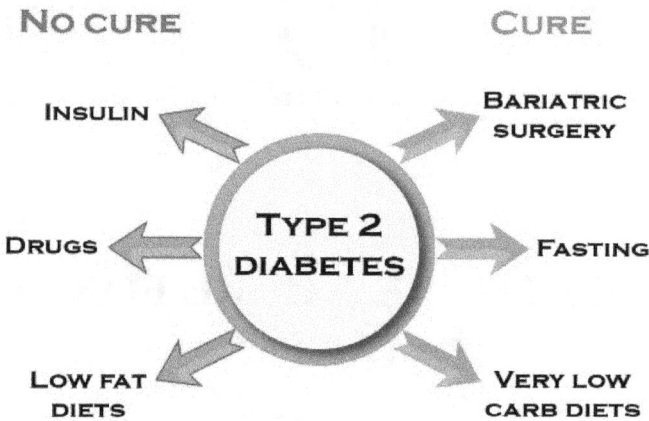

Fig. 22: Changing concepts for 'curing' Type 2 Diabetes.

Type-2 diabetes is not a disease per se, but an altered physiological response or adaptation by the body. It is not a disease because there is nothing broken or missing. The pancreas is still making insulin. But it is not being used optimally. Our body is a smart system designed to have a balance or homeostasis. When things get out of balance in the body, it is because something is making it go out of balance.

The body will always attempt to return to homeostasis as soon as the instigating factor is gone. Your body is designed to do the right thing for the right reasons. Let us look at a few examples to help you understand this better.

What is hypertrophy? It is when something grows larger. A bodybuilder uses heavy weights and exerts his muscles repeatedly, many times or many hours a day. The resultant growing of muscle or hypertrophy is an adaptation of the body to an imposed demand. We have pushed the muscle and the muscle responds. The opposite or atrophy happens when muscles don't have any activity, like in someone who has broken a limb or is paralyzed. If you don't use the muscle for anything, the body will downsize or down-regulate it as it doesn't want to spend precious resources rebuilding that muscle if it's not going to be used. Everything the body does is in response to a requirement. This is called physiological adaptation.

Diabetes is a late-stage result of insulin resistance. When we eat things that trigger insulin, primarily sugar and carbohydrates, the insulin production goes up. If we do this six times a day, then insulin production goes up six times a day and starts pushing blood sugar into the cell. When the cell has had enough fuel, it starts resisting and starts adapting. With more and more fuel coming, the cell adapts and stops taking in the excess fuel. When the body is overwhelmed, it is going to try to oppose that factor and become insulin resistant until that avalanche of fuel and sugar starts to pull back. High blood sugar or diabetes are imbalances that develop over time because we are pushing the body and the body is adapting to respond. Hence, type-2 diabetes is not a disease but a physiological adaptation or the body's intelligent response to an unbalanced environment. The unbalanced environment is modern food; it's the carbohydrates and sugar and processed foods in amounts that the human body has never experienced.

Rather than understanding the body's innate intelligence and homeostasis, we believe that the body breaks down for no reason, which is not true. We think of insulin resistance as cells that are no longer responding normally to blood glucose or to normal food anymore. A normal diet today has close to 300 grams of carbohydrates, in the form of sugar and starches. We have to first put the body back on meals that are normal for humans and what we had been eating for the longest time before junk and processed food entered the picture. This is a crucial factor in the understanding of holistic health. We need to reduce or reverse the factors that force the physiological adaptation in diabetes. We need to eat less of the food that stimulates insulin, such as sugars, processed food, and any kind of starch, especially processed starches. If you are already insulin resistant, eat less sugar, moderate to very little fruit, and cut out grains (both processed and complex). Eat less frequently because when you eat something it stimulates insulin. Each time you eat, you get one burst of insulin. If you eat six times, you are pushing insulin six times and you are giving the cells six more chances to become insulin resistant. The longer the gap between meals, the greater the opportunity for the cell to start burning some of that fuel.

Don't wait for a type-2 diabetes cure. We need to understand that a cure is a healing process or a reversal of the adaptation. There is never going to be a pill that can cure or fix the homeostasis because the body is always intelligent and will adapt to the imbalance. And if you have created that imbalance, just take remedial measures and your body will go right back to doing what it's supposed to do.

"Every form of addiction is bad; be it drugs or food. Whatever it may be, too much is always too bad!"

13

LOW CARB HEALTHY FAT DIET –WHAT YOU NEED TO KNOW

"You may have to fight a battle more than once to win it."
Margaret Thatcher

Since the 1960s, doctors have been advising us to avoid saturated fat to prevent heart disease, but recent evidence shows the contrary. In the 1970s, dietary guidelines specifically recommended us to avoid eating too much fat and cholesterol but the evidence to support this statement was not very strong. It was based on a few observations that showed an association between countries that ate a lot of saturated fat and their rate of heart disease.

However, that correlation was very weak and recommendations were made hastily to avoid fat. This led to a change in habits from eating animal fats like butter, which are high in saturated fats, to being replaced with unsaturated fats or hydrogenated vegetable oils. If we look at the science behind this, we will see that the amount of saturated fat in our blood is more related to the amount of carbohydrate intake. Through the process of lipogenesis, the excess carbohydrates are converted into fats for storage. Though the reason behind the low-fat diet was to reduce heart disease and lower the LDL cholesterol, newer research has shown that it is not quite that simple.

Lower fat diets tend to reduce the larger LDL particles, which are not thought to cause heart disease. In fact, an article published in the journal of the American College of Cardiology in August 2020 found that people who ate more fat tended to be protected against strokes. Whole fat dairy, red meat and dark chocolate, which are complex food matrices, have a lot of saturated fat.

Specialists suggest that we should make recommendations not on specific nutrients but base them on whole foods. We shouldn't be avoiding fat because we don't eat plain 'fat' - we eat dairy and meat which are whole foods. Increased carbohydrates in the diet increases the amount of saturated fat in the blood.

Food is more than just the macronutrients it contains - the carbs, the proteins and the fats - because there are differences between the types of fats that are in it. The interaction between the naturally occurring and the unhealthy components which are induced by food processing is most important.

In the 1950s, vegetable oils were recognized to lower our serum cholesterol and therefore thought to be heart healthy. This led to a huge movement away from butter and we were encouraged to eat more vegetable oils, which were hydrogenated thereby creating trans fats. Subsequent research in the 1980s and 1990s showed that these trans fats are the reason for heart diseases.

In 1997, a very large study showed that the fat you ate is not related to the risk of heart disease and in 2001, top researchers reported that it is increasingly recognized that the low-fat campaign had been based on little scientific evidence and may have caused unintended health consequences. We are starting to see that foods high in fat like nuts, avocados and olive oil are really not unhealthy. Eating more saturated fat is actually protective against heart disease and stroke according to a study on 58,000 people who were divided into five different groups. The group that ate the most saturated fat had an adjusted odds ratio of about 0.7 to 0.8, meaning they had 20 to 30 percent less risk of heart disease, stroke and mortality compared to those who ate the least saturated fat. This is also proven by the fact that the French had a lot less heart disease compared to other countries in the 1980s and 1990s, when they ate a lot of whole fat dairy.

More recently, in 2017, a large epidemiologic study was published in the Lancet, which covered 18 countries and 135000 people who were followed up over seven years. Saturated fat, total fat and carbohydrates consumed by them was monitored and compared to the rates of heart disease. They found that the risk of heart disease tended to go down as more saturated fat was consumed. A higher percentage of carbohydrates in the diet showed a higher risk of heart disease.

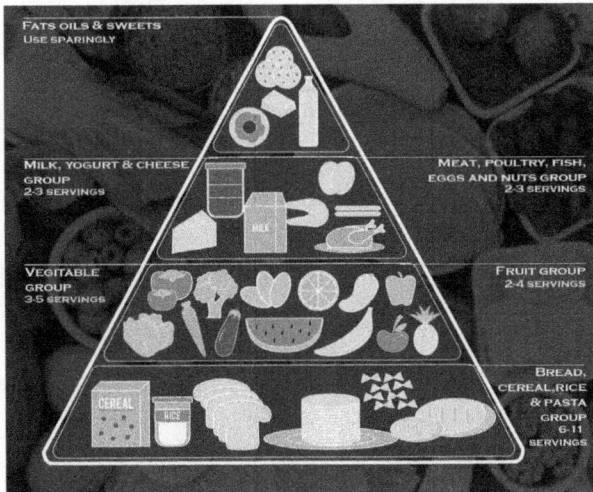

Fig. 23: Classical teaching food pyramid.

Eating more natural saturated fats is recommended, as in a keto diet. You can eat full-fat cheese and full-fat milk without an increased risk of heart disease or diabetes and it will also be protective against strokes and facilitate weight loss. Coming to the benefits of a low-carb, healthy-fat (LCHF) diet, the first is a reduction in hunger because there are no spikes in the blood glucose levels, which are far more constant. Adopting an LCHF diet will give diabetics better glucose control and most likely lead to a reduction in the amount of insulin required.

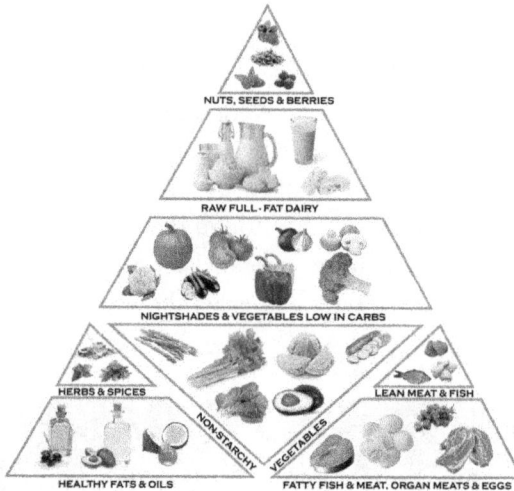

Fig. 24: Low-carb-High fat food pyramid.

An LCHF diet also results in a significant decrease in triglycerides and an increase in HDL or good cholesterol. Total and LDL cholesterol usually remain about the same. It results in increased particle size which has been associated with reduced risk of cardiovascular disease. Many people feel that their gastrointestinal symptoms such as abdominal discomfort and bloating are reduced. Restricting carbohydrates during childhood also helps prevent childhood obesity, which frequently leads to adult obesity. Childhood diseases such as attention deficit hyperactivity disorder or ADHD have also been linked to excessive carbohydrates, especially sugar intake.

An endurance athlete can perform just as well with an LCHF diet, if not better, as fat is a very efficient fuel and, unlike carbohydrate, there is no limit to its stores.

It is best to eat natural foods and avoid processed foods.

There are lots of enjoyable, tasty foods that are suitable for an LCHF diet such as eggs, meat, dairy and green vegetables, so sustaining the diet is not a problem.

You can eat as many vegetables that grow above the ground as you like, such as cauliflower, broccoli, cabbage, Brussels sprouts, asparagus, zucchini, eggplant, olives, spinach, mushrooms, cucumber, lettuce, avocado, onions, peppers, and tomatoes. Eat healthy fats from avocado and nuts such as almonds, walnuts, Brazil nuts, hazelnuts, and macadamia nuts.

Cook with healthy oils and fats like butter, olive oil, and coconut oil. Berries such as strawberries, raspberries, blackberries, and blueberries are the most suitable fruit. You can also have dairy like full fat milk, cream, butter, cheese, and Greek yogurt. Drink as much as you want of water, herb tea, black coffee, and green tea.

You can eat a moderate amount of the best quality protein that you can get - a mixture of red and white meat (preferably pasture fed, not grain fed), fish, and eggs. Cut back on sugar from soft drinks, candy, juice, sports drinks, chocolate, cakes, buns, pastries, and ice cream. Avoid bread and related products like biscuits, muffins, and cakes. Cut down on breakfast cereals, rice, potatoes, and other starchy vegetables. Most fruit (except berries) contain a large amount of fructose – a carbohydrate even more harmful than glucose. Avoid fruit juices which are full of sugar, flavored yogurts, and beer.

Do not cook with vegetable or seed oils such as canola, sunflower, and safflower oil. You can occasionally drink alcohol – red or white wine, and spirits, and eat chocolate with 70% cocoa. With these modifications, your health and life will be back on track in no time!

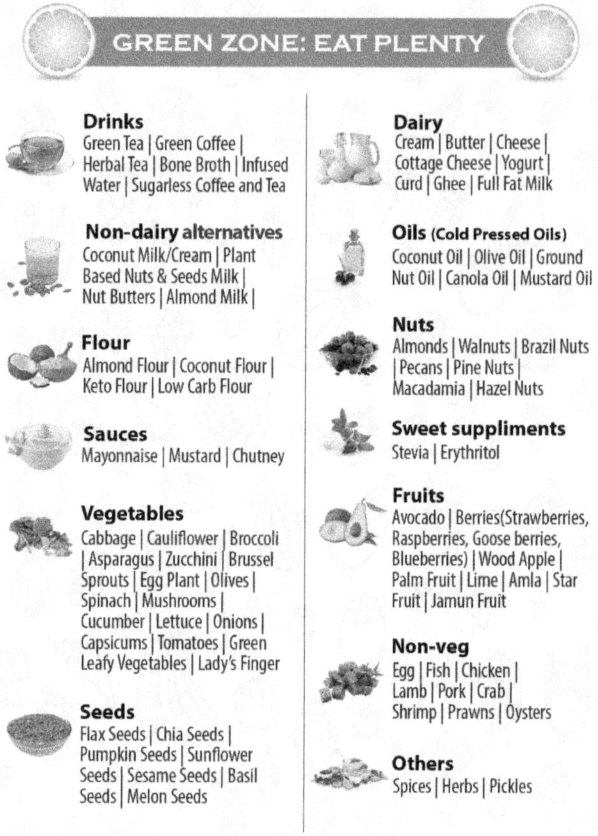

GREEN ZONE: EAT PLENTY

Drinks
Green Tea | Green Coffee | Herbal Tea | Bone Broth | Infused Water | Sugarless Coffee and Tea

Non-dairy alternatives
Coconut Milk/Cream | Plant Based Nuts & Seeds Milk | Nut Butters | Almond Milk |

Flour
Almond Flour | Coconut Flour | Keto Flour | Low Carb Flour

Sauces
Mayonnaise | Mustard | Chutney

Vegetables
Cabbage | Cauliflower | Broccoli | Asparagus | Zucchini | Brussel Sprouts | Egg Plant | Olives | Spinach | Mushrooms | Cucumber | Lettuce | Onions | Capsicums | Tomatoes | Green Leafy Vegetables | Lady's Finger

Seeds
Flax Seeds | Chia Seeds | Pumpkin Seeds | Sunflower Seeds | Sesame Seeds | Basil Seeds | Melon Seeds

Dairy
Cream | Butter | Cheese | Cottage Cheese | Yogurt | Curd | Ghee | Full Fat Milk

Oils (Cold Pressed Oils)
Coconut Oil | Olive Oil | Ground Nut Oil | Canola Oil | Mustard Oil

Nuts
Almonds | Walnuts | Brazil Nuts | Pecans | Pine Nuts | Macadamia | Hazel Nuts

Sweet suppliments
Stevia | Erythritol

Fruits
Avocado | Berries(Strawberries, Raspberries, Goose berries, Blueberries) | Wood Apple | Palm Fruit | Lime | Amla | Star Fruit | Jamun Fruit

Non-veg
Egg | Fish | Chicken | Lamb | Pork | Crab | Shrimp | Prawns | Oysters

Others
Spices | Herbs | Pickles

Fig 25: Foods safe to consume

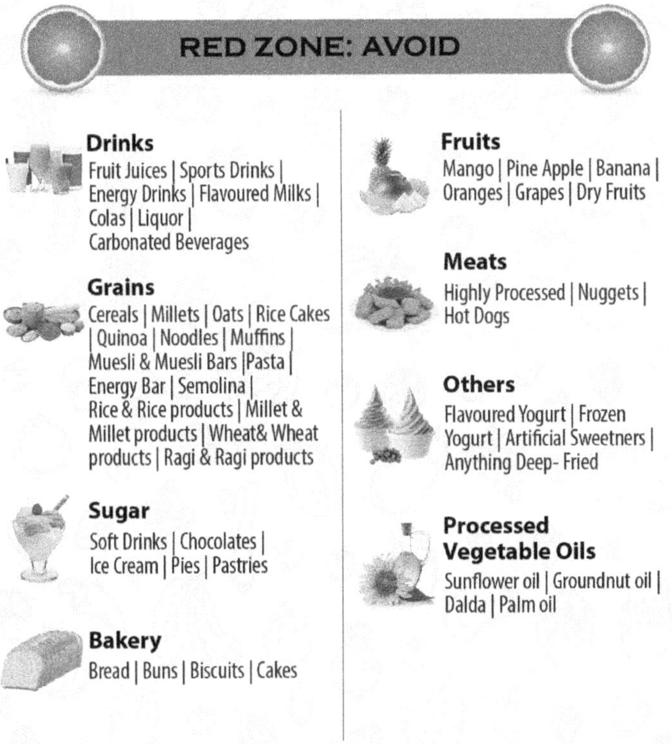

RED ZONE: AVOID

Drinks
Fruit Juices | Sports Drinks | Energy Drinks | Flavoured Milks | Colas | Liquor | Carbonated Beverages

Grains
Cereals | Millets | Oats | Rice Cakes | Quinoa | Noodles | Muffins | Muesli & Muesli Bars |Pasta | Energy Bar | Semolina | Rice & Rice products | Millet & Millet products | Wheat& Wheat products | Ragi & Ragi products

Sugar
Soft Drinks | Chocolates | Ice Cream | Pies | Pastries

Bakery
Bread | Buns | Biscuits | Cakes

Fruits
Mango | Pine Apple | Banana | Oranges | Grapes | Dry Fruits

Meats
Highly Processed | Nuggets | Hot Dogs

Others
Flavoured Yogurt | Frozen Yogurt | Artificial Sweetners | Anything Deep- Fried

Processed Vegetable Oils
Sunflower oil | Groundnut oil | Dalda | Palm oil

Fig. 26: Foods to avoid

14

INTERMITTENT FASTING – THE NEW MANTRA!

"Eat when hungry, stop when full, never eat by the clock"

Before we look at intermittent fasting, let us first understand what fasting is? Fasting is simply "when you don't eat." If you eat every two hours, you are fasting for two hours, and if you eat every four hours, you are fasting for four hours. A lot of people equate fasting with starving, which is not true. We have been told to eat these many meals a day, failing which we will get sick. When one goes longer without food, there is a sensation of hunger. Hunger is a natural instinct and your body's way of telling you that it wants some food. This is where your carb dependency comes in.

Intermittent fasting is simply the period of time between meals. It is not a diet but a pattern of eating. In fact, almost all of us are already doing it. If you eat breakfast in the morning, lunch at noon, a snack at 3:00 pm, have dinner late evening, and a bedtime snack or fruit, you will have had a 3 hour fast throughout the day between each meal. If you do not eat during the night, you have a 12 hour fast between the last meal and the first meal of the next day. So, all of us are already doing around 12 hours of intermittent fasting while we sleep at night. We are able to survive this because the body has mechanisms or systems to compensate and maintain stability during the fasting period. People on intermittent fasting eat whatever they are already eating, but will skip a meal to get a longer fasting period and this will help them become healthier.

A lot of people think that intermittent fasting is a trend or a fad, but this practice has been around for centuries. Most races around the world have had an element of fasting built into religious or cultural traditions. Importantly, our ancestors did not wake up to a breakfast buffet and never had three meals a day, much less six. They probably ate one or two substantial meals a day when they were able to find it (fruits), hunt for it (meat), or produce it (grain). In between they might have snacked on some berries or some nuts, if and when available. They did not have ways to preserve food such as refrigerators and freezers to make abundant food available at all times. If they were unable to find food, they ended up fasting for variable periods of time. Their blood sugars probably remained stable because they did not have a significant amount of carbohydrates or an abundance of processed and starchy foods or frequent meals. So, whatever our ancestors developed and adapted to, can also work for us.

The benefits of intermittent fasting are endless. People who could never reduce insulin resistance or weight are able to do so relatively easily by switching to intermittent fasting. It can lower LDL levels (a marker of inflammation) and increase HDL levels and reverse conditions such as cardiovascular disease and diabetes, which are often considered incurable. These conditions are not really a disease in the first place but an adaptation of the body. Even the probability of developing cancer can be greatly reduced. Longer periods of fasting can induce "autophagy", which is a very powerful healing and anti-aging tool which recycles and cleans up the body's resources and rebuilds things.

Those who do not approve of intermittent fasting typically say things like "breakfast is the most important meal of the day or that you should eat small but frequent meals or that if you don't eat often enough your blood sugar is going to drop". These things are true only if your body is adapted to or dependent on a high carbohydrate diet or frequent meals. This creates a blood sugar rollercoaster which goes up and down every time you eat and it's these rapid swings that create health issues.

Given a chance, our body can adapt very well to skipping a meal. It has plenty of mechanisms to generate energy, manage, and stabilize blood sugar and energy levels in the absence of food. However, it has no defense against six meals a day and does not know what to do with the excess food (energy) that we keep consuming. This is why we develop lifestyle diseases and intermittent fasting can help reverse them. When you eat, you trigger insulin which is a fat storage hormone. So, every time you eat, you are telling your body to store something. If you eat six meals a day or a lot of carbohydrates, insulin is going to put the sugar out of the bloodstream and into the cell. The cell will use some of it and will store the rest as fat. A constantly high insulin level is going to prevent you from retrieving that stored fat and using it for fuel. Even if you eat small frequent meals, you have an insulin response every time that you eat and you are building up your insulin resistance.

Most people do not realize the number of meals they have in a day - all the little snacks such as a small bite of a cake, or a biscuit or an energy bar, a little sip of fruit juice or a mug of tea or coffee – can be over 15 times per day. This will in turn trigger blood sugar and insulin. If we don't consume sugar and carbs so often, the body will learn to adapt in between. The longer you go in between meals, the body has a higher chance at finding fuel elsewhere than what you are eating.

All of us walk around with at least a hundred thousand calories of fat in our bodies. The key reason that intermittent fasting works is that once you go longer between meals it allows you to be calorie deficit without getting hungry if you are fat-adapted.

While intermittent fasting is more popular to lose weight, it can also turn around insulin resistance, which is the primary factor responsible for obesity, diabetes, cardiovascular disease, stroke, dementia, and auto immune diseases. For people who find it hard to start or stick to skipping meals for hours or days at a time, these following tips can simplify the process and help make the transition easy and effortless.

The first is to understand that you are already doing intermittent fasting. If you eat your dinner at 9:00 pm and have your breakfast at 8:00 am, you have been fasting for 11 hours, unless you had a midnight snack. Your body can survive the night because it has adapted to being without food for those 11-12 hours.

Now, all you need to do is to train your body to manage longer periods of fasting during the waking hours. Easiest way is to eliminate all the in-between snacks, so that you have only 3 meals a day.

Next is to start reducing the carbohydrate intake. If you are eating 300 grams of carbs a day, gradually work your way down to maybe 100 grams. As you do this, you are going to notice that you get less and less hungry but it's going to take a while for your body to change its machinery around and learn how to use fat. Just work your way down until you are less hungry and you are more stable. Once you are on a lower carb diet you will have less swings of blood sugar and it will not impact you much if you skip a meal.

When you cut back the carbs, you have to replace it with something. The thing that triggers insulin the least is fat. So, eat the good fats and things that naturally have good fat in them. This includes avocado and nuts, meat from grass-fed animals, butter, olive oil, and coconut oil. You can also supplement your meals with some green leafy vegetables.

Once you start adapting, you can increase your fasting window further. Instead of having dinner at 9:00 pm you can have it at 6:00

pm and don't have anything afterwards. You can start increasing it even further by having breakfast a little bit later. You can have brunch at noon and dinner at 6:00 pm giving you an 18-hour fasting window. Your period of fasting is three times longer than your period of eating and this is a tremendously powerful tool to reduce insulin. Now you are going much longer without insulin which gives your body the time to become more insulin sensitive. Eat only when you are really hungry. We often eat just because 'it is meal time' or due to cravings or because it's a habit.

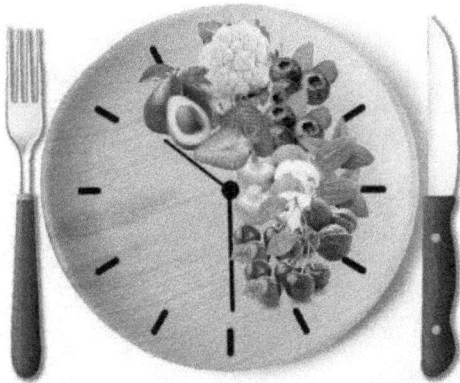

Fig. 27: Customize your eating and fasting window.

For the most part, you can ignore the tiny little rumblings or hunger pangs. A cup of green tea can easily make it go away. But if you get really hungry, then it's ok to eat. Plan ahead and make sure that you have some good food available. If there is no healthy food around, you will end up eating some junk or processed food. Healthy snacks include cheese or nuts. Now that you understand how easy it is, you can consider making the switch to intermittent fasting. Besides helping with reversing insulin resistance, it also helps in weight management. There are lots of ways to lose weight in an unhealthy way and there are lots of skinny people who are very unhealthy. Since skinny people can also get diabetes, high blood pressure and cancer, we can't just jump to the conclusion that the extra weight is the cause of the bad health. We have to understand that the excess weight is not the cause but the result of an unhealthy lifestyle and weight loss is not proof of health.

While intermittent fasting is safe for most people, pregnant women and breastfeeding mothers, people who are underweight, children and teenagers in the developmental age group, should avoid it since intermittent fasting causes a calorie deficit. Intermittent fasting should also not be considered a rapid or short gap solution. Nature has a certain pace; if it took you a certain amount of time to gain weight or develop insulin resistance, it is going to take a while to turn it around.

WHAT ARE THE BENEFITS OF INTERMITTENT FASTING?

FAT BURNING	POTENTIAL TREATMENT OR EVEN REVERSAL OF TYPE 2 DIABETES
IMPROVED MENTAL CLARITY AND CONCENTRATION	ANTI-AGING BENEFITS
LOWERED BLOOD SUGAR AND INSULIN LEVELS	MAY PREVENT CANCER AND REDUCE THE SIDE EFFECTS OF CANCER
INCREASED ENERGY	IMPROVED IMMUNE SYSTEM
LOWERS RISKS OF HEART DISEASE	REDUCES BAD CHOLESTEROL LEVELS
WEIGHT LOSS	CELLULAR REPAIR, WHICH MAY PROVIDE PROTECTION AGAINST SEVERAL DISEASES
REGULATES BLOOD PRESSURE	REDUCES OXIDATIVE STRESS AND INFLAMMATION IN THE BODY

Fig. 28: Benefits of intermittent fasting

The body has to rebuild and regenerate in the right way. You can lose some weight quickly, but that is not healthy. Health is when every cell and every organ in your body is functioning optimally. If you want to get healthy then you have to get your cells and your organs healthy, and you have to provide them with good nutrients. If you keep eating processed foods, junk food, and frequent meals, or lots and lots of carbohydrate and sugar, you are upsetting the balance in the body. Intermittent fasting is a lifestyle change that can help fight lifestyle diseases. It is a change that does not cost much, is easy to implement, and has long lasting health benefits.

"Intermittent fasting is incredibly useful in aiding fat loss, preventing cancer, building muscle, and increasing resilience. Done correctly, it's one of the most painless high-impact ways to live longer."
- Dave Asprey

15

STRESS AND DIABETES

"Stress exacerbates any problem, whether it's diabetes, heart trouble, multiple sclerosis, or whatever."
Mary Ann Mobley

Stress is an underlying cause for several health problems and can also contribute to the development of diabetes. While diet, weight and exercise, are frequently spoken about, 'stress' is rarely discussed. It is a feeling of being overwhelmed or frustrated. A feeling of helplessness when multiple things are going on at the same time and we cannot keep up. Like we have 'bitten off more than we can chew'! And all this could just be the tip of the iceberg, with several other stressors being unknown or undetected. This stress can increase the demand on our body's physiological reaction - our adrenal glands release adrenaline, our heart rate goes up, we clench our jaws, the blood pressure goes up, there is an increase in the muscle tone, an upregulation of low-density lipoprotein cholesterol, to name a few. Any acute stressor, be it a physical trauma or an emotional one or a chemical trauma like chemotherapy or toxicity, induces a physiological response to trigger the sympathetic nervous system. All these require more energy, which means more blood sugar and cortisol, which also in turn trigger more insulin.

Most often, the physiological and physical responses go completely unnoticed either because we are not paying attention or because we are so used to it or it has been that way for too long. Chronic stress leads to a sympathetic dominance when we tend to produce cortisol at a higher level and for longer periods of time leading to a higher baseline activity.

Studies on healthy people who are insulin sensitive but injected with cortisol have shown measurable changes in the insulin resistance within days.

Many people treated with systemic steroids for inflammatory diseases develop raised blood sugars, higher insulin and a definite risk for insulin resistance and weight gain.

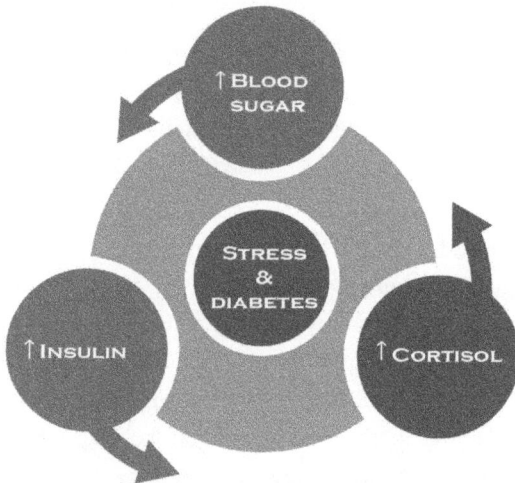

Fig. 29: The Stress and Diabetes Loop

Elizabeth Blackburn, an Australian-American scientist, was

awarded the Nobel Prize in 2009 for having discovered that 'telomeres' prevent chromosomes from being broken down in 1980. What are 'telomeres' and how do they affect our lives? Simply put, these are complex structures at the end of our chromosomes that protect them from deterioration. They are like the little erasers at the end of the pencils or like the plastic tips of shoelaces. Over time these either wear out or become too short to function optimally.

So is the case with telomeres. In many ways, telomeres act as 'ageing clocks' in every cell. They are important for our general well-being. An enzyme called 'telomerase' helps in increasing the telomere's length and increases the longevity of the telomere and extends its function. Telomerase is *decreased* by stress and nutritional deficiency and *increased* by good nutrition, regular exercise, less stress and a positive outlook. If you are engaging in 'telomerase-increasing' activities, you are protecting yourself from disease and disability. There is substantial scientific correlation between health and a stress-free life.

When we face a situation that is potentially stressful, it is our mind that interprets the environment and the situation. Our perception is critical. We are not the victim of our genes but the masters of them. Can stress cause diabetes? We know that cortisol raises blood sugar, which can drive insulin resistance, but can it really cause diabetes in itself? It is unlikely that diabetes results if the only problem is stress. But with a majority of the population already having some degree of insulin resistance, stress becomes a very significant contributory factor.

We also need to consider lifestyle factors, diet, genetics, and physical activity as major contributors. If you have one or more of these risks, then stress can push you over the edge. If you are pre-diabetic, consume lots of carbohydrates and lead a sedentary lifestyle, stress can push you further into becoming a diabetic. Addressing only one of the factors is not adequate to reduce your overall risk.

Reducing stress is easier said than done. Identifying the cause and aggravators is important. Self-help or professional help is a call you need to take. Regular sleep, meditation, relaxation, and deep breathing exercises are some habits to inculcate. When we are in a positive frame of mind, hormones like dopamine and oxytocin are released, which give us the feeling of well-being and happiness. Ninety percent of all lifestyle diseases are related to stress. The trick here is to train the mind to be positive in all circumstances. Try to find the silver lining in every dark cloud. If you have your mind under your control, you will have the world at your feet. You also need to understand that your mind is governed by how healthy your body is. If you are fat adapted with a low carb lifestyle, your blood sugar will remain more stable which will help to balance out the stress-induced cortisol that has an influence on blood sugar. With several contributing factors to the risk of diabetes, adapting to a low carb diet may offer some help in these 'stressful' times!

"To keep the body in good health is a duty, otherwise we shall not be able to keep our mind strong and clear."
-Buddha

16

PLEASURE TRAP

"A journey of a thousand miles begins with a single step."
Lao Tzu

Douglas J. Lisle, Professor of Public Health Sciences and Psychiatry at Penn State University in the U.S., speaks about 'The Motivational Triad': the search for pleasure, pain-prevention, and conservation of the energy.

Humans have "magic buttons," as Dr. Lisle calls them - drugs, gambling, and food. These magic buttons are dangerous as they attract the instincts embedded in the triad of motivation, but steal victims of happiness and health.

This disappointment is called the 'pleasure trap', which is the insidious force or the internal compass of your nervous system, telling you what's best for you.

One of the most destructive elements of the pleasure trap is food. Some studies speculate that this might be the result of improper functioning of neuronal circuits and have shown that obese subjects might have an impairment in the dopaminergic pathways that regulate neuronal systems associated with reward sensitivity, conditioning, and control.

When we engage in pleasurable activities, our brain starts secreting a chemical called dopamine, which is the same dependent neurotransmitter associated with alcohol, smoking or drug addiction.

Though there is a disturbing picture of the adverse effects of cancer on cigarette packets, it hasn't deterred people. Likewise, despite labels on food products listing out the high amounts of sugar in the ingredients, we still eat them as they are so delicious. Let us look at the phases of the Pleasure Trap:

Phase I:

We give in to our desires and end up having a few cheat meals. But everything is still under control in this phase.

Phase II:

In the second phase, unnatural or processed foods have a negative influence on our system, like a drug. Our body starts getting used to the excessive use of sugar and grains in our diets owing to the delicious taste.

Phase III:

In the third phase, the unnatural food that we have got used to controls us. Even though we know all the harmful outcomes, it is difficult for us to resist.

Phase IV:

Switching to a healthy diet give us subnormal pleasure. At this phase, many find it difficult and give up.

Phase V:

Those who persist for 4-6 weeks on a healthy diet move from sub-normal pleasure to normalcy.

The Pleasure Trap – it's all in the mind!

Tips to Avoid the Pleasure Trap:

- Plan ahead
- Eat consciously
- Give your palate time to adjust
- Read some books, do some research and watch a few relatable videos.

One of the most destructive elements of the pleasure trap is food. Life is short, so don't waste it by giving in to your pleasures. Learn to control your mind and prioritize things. In the end, it is all in your hands. If you set your mind on something, don't stop until you reach that goal. Accept that it's going to be hard, but important. Your system will then reboot and adapt to the new diet if you persist.

Your health is in your mouth.
Control what goes into it for physical health.
Control what comes out of it for mental health.

17

LET FOOD BE THY MEDICINE

"Genetics only load the gun, but it is the environment that pulls the trigger."
— Francis Collins

After a full-fledged battle against tobacco, it is now time for us to wage a war against bad dietary habits. It took 35 years and more than 7,000 research papers to understand the ill-effects of smoking. We all learnt it the hard way.

HEALTH SPAN VS. LIFE SPAN

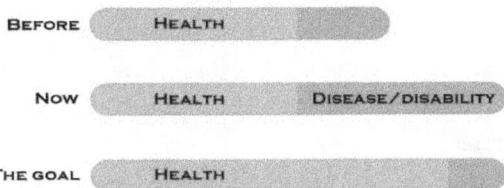

BEFORE	HEALTH	
NOW	HEALTH	DISEASE/DISABILITY
THE GOAL	HEALTH	

Fig. 30: Relation between health and disease with life span

However, bad habits are not easy to break. Despite all the awareness that has been created, people still smoke, bringing harm to themselves and the people around them. **As our lifespan increases, our health quotient should increase proportionately.**

Everything changes if you start looking at food as something that influences our immune system. An unhealthy diet could cause incalculable damage to our health. While we cannot control everything in life, the food we consume is completely under our control. There will be barriers [beliefs, opinions, assumptions, traditions, cultures], but if you want a long and healthy life, then take a step towards bettering it today! Take it step by step — one day at a time.

Prevention is always better than cure. Instead of consulting a doctor after things go out of hand, take preventive measures before you fall ill. Start by looking for some easy-to-prepare low carbs healthy fat recipes, and choose ingredients and flavors that you and your family relish. The key is to focus on eating for the betterment of your health. A healthy diet offers many of the healthy nutrients you need, including omega-3 fatty acids, fibers, antioxidants, various minerals and vitamins, which have significant health benefits. The World Health Organization says that it is never too late to start eating better and people who followed a healthy dietary pattern saw a two-year rise in life expectancy.

Food plays a social and ceremonial role in many cultures, and has a cultural connotation for many, with vegetarian and non-vegetarian diet being preferred by different sections of the society. This is very evident, especially in countries like India, which has so many cultures and traditions. '*Atithi Devo Bhava*' is something Indians follow. We never send a guest back without offering food, and sometimes tend to even force-feed them. Overzealous Indian mothers tend to overfeed their children without realizing the harm it can do to them in the long run.

Hippocrates, the Father of Medicine, once said, "Let food be thy medicine and medicine be thy food," indicating that a healthy diet plays a major role in the prevention of lifestyle diseases. On the contrary, food addiction is a lifestyle disease demonstrated by the fact that we constantly crave food, eat compulsively, and find it difficult to control these urges despite being aware of the adverse consequences. But the power is within you to make a healthy choice, and you should be determined to achieve it and not stop until the goal is reached.

A young man once asked Socrates about the secret to success. Socrates, being a wise man, asked the young man to meet him near the river the next morning if he wanted to find the answer. Next morning, both started walking by the river and then towards the river, and finally found themselves inside the river. Socrates suddenly ducked the young man's face into the water. The young man struggled to free himself from Socrates's hand; however, he could not.

Socrates finally pulled him up, and the young man gasped and took a deep breath of air. "What did you want the most when your head was in the water?" Socrates asked the young man, to which he replied, saying "Air, of course."

Socrates smiled and said, "That is the secret to success. When you want success as badly as you wanted the air while you were in the water, you will get it. There is no other secret." If you want something in life, instead of looking for answers on the outside, look right inside of you.

Introspect and ask yourself what is it that you want and work towards it.

So How Exactly Does Food Work Like Medicine? Take A Look at This:

1. Consume food items that decrease inflammation. It is told that antioxidants protect cells from damage that may otherwise lead to disease. Cruciferous vegetables like broccoli, brussels sprouts, and green leafy vegetables provide our body with a wide array of antioxidants. They

help fight against heart disease and other chronic conditions.

2. Eating right also helps balance hormones, alkalizes the body, and helps maintain blood sugar levels. An LCHF diet cleanses the body by eliminating toxins.

3. Foods that are rich in fiber not only facilitate proper digestion but also feed the good bacteria in your gut.

4. Studies have also revealed that a diet rich in berries may protect you against chronic conditions, including certain cancers.

5. Spices like turmeric, ginger, and cinnamon have proven positive effects on conditions like arthritis.

6. At least 50-60% of your diet should be in the form of vegetables in each meal.

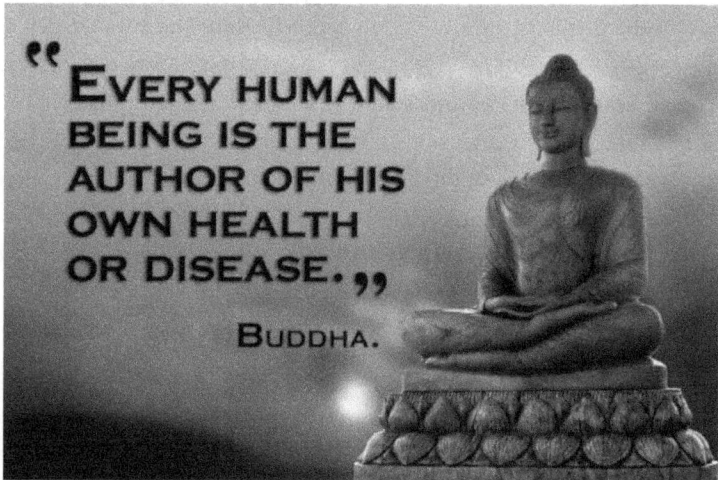

Taking the onus

"The primary duty of a doctor is not to treat the sick, but to prevent sickness"

18

KEEP A TAB TO KEEP THE TABS
AT BAY!

A Continuous Glucose Monitor (CGM) is a wearable biosensor which helps you monitor and manage Type I and Type 2 diabetes in a better way. A sensor on the skin measures your glucose levels 24 hours a day in real time. Your blood sugars are affected by many things including the food you eat, physical activity, stress, and sleep. We know that diabetes affects everyone differently and similarly diet and exercise can variably alter glucose levels. This is where a CGM helps. It keeps a tab on your sugar levels throughout the day and it becomes easy to determine which food item or workout has the maximum effect – good or bad! While a finger prick test gives you blood glucose levels at that moment, a CGM periodically assesses the sugar levels in the interstitial fluid. Hence, it is not an actual measure of blood sugar but rather the glucose that continuously oozes from the blood vessels and capillaries into this fluid. You can calibrate your CGM with a glucometer test to improve the accuracy. While this device is surely helpful for diabetics, it can help all of us understand how diet and lifestyle decisions affect our health and to ensure stable glucose levels before metabolic dysfunction like insulin resistance or prediabetes sets in.

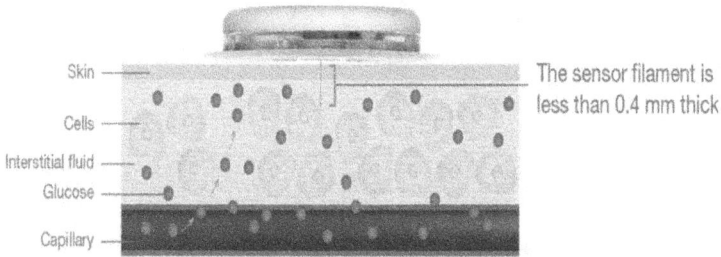

For illustrative purposes only. Image not drawn to scale.

Fig. 31: Continuous Glucose Monitor (CGM)
Source: Abbott

A CGM is a round plastic device that typically sticks to the skin of your upper arm or stomach. It sends glucose data continuously to your smartphone or handheld device at least every 5 minutes. Below the plastic disc is a flexible 5mm long and 0.4mm wide filament. When the CGM is applied to your skin, a small spring-loaded needle guides this filament through your skin painlessly, leaving the end of the filament in the interstitial fluid just below the skin.

The device wirelessly transmits data, which is presented as a graph or chart using an algorithm in your smartphone. Without a CGM, the only way to closely monitor blood sugars and adjust your medicine dosage is to use a glucometer dozens of times a day. If your blood sugar gets too high, there is an option to connect the CGM to an insulin pump to automatically deliver insulin to your body.

Most CGMs last for one to two weeks before they need replacement. There are newer devices in the pipeline offering more features, including optional real-time alarms to alert you when glucose levels get too high or too low.

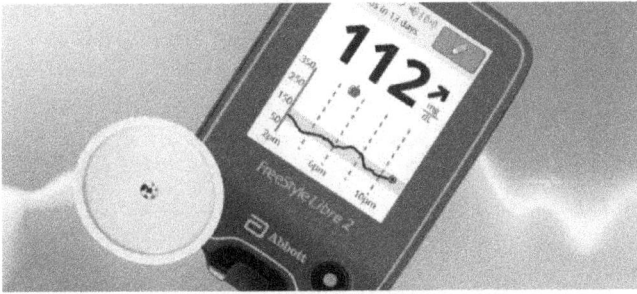

Fig. 32: Readings from the Continuous Glucose Monitor (CGM)
(Source: Abbott)

While fasting blood glucose and HbA1c assessments are accurate, they provide only a single measurement, at a particular time point. They do not show how much your blood sugar is spiking and crashing - the glycemic variability or roller coaster. They do not give information about trends over time or reactions to particular foods or activities.

For diabetics, high or low blood sugar can be life-threatening. Consistently high glucose levels can damage the vessels that supply blood to vital organs, increase the risk of heart disease and stroke, kidney disease, vision issues, nerve problems, and lead to fatigue, brain fog, and depression. Low blood sugar or hypoglycemia leads to symptoms like sweating, palpitations, dizziness, tiredness, hunger, and irritability.

Hence, good monitoring and management of glucose

greatly helps people with diabetes stay healthy and prevent complications with improved quality of life.

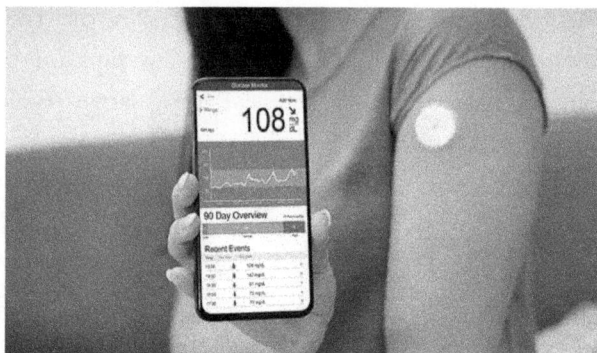

Fig. 33: Mobile apps to Continuously Monitor Sugars

To summarize, a CGM helps to:

- Tailor your diet to avoid glucose spikes
- Titrate your medication to avoid hypoglycemia
- Monitor glycemic load and glycemic response
- Avoid foods spiking sugars – grains, potatoes
- Pair less ripe fruits with fat and protein to optimize blood glucose
- Experiment with different foods to check your response
- Plan timing of food or eating window
- Prevent the glucose level roller coaster
- Make yourself more metabolically flexible
- Detect metabolic dysfunction early

19

COMMON QUESTIONS – SIMPLE ANSWERS!

1. What is the difference between Keto and Low Carb diet?

Keto – stands for ketosis – which is a metabolic state wherein the body make ketones from fats and uses it as fuel instead of the normally used glucose for energy. For the body to get into ketosis, we need to reduce the intake of sugar and carbs to less than 50gm per day.

LCHF is a well formulated low carb healthy fat diet. How low to go on the carbs will depend from person to person and their goals, be it losing weight or reversing diabetes.

2. What is an LCHF diet?

LCHF stands for a Low Carb Healthy Fat diet. It typically contains

70 to 75 per cent healthy fat, 20 per cent protein, and about 5 to 10 per cent carbs. In terms of grams per day, it would be:

- 20-50g of carbohydrate
- 60-80g of protein
- A good portion of healthy or good fats

Fats in the diet provide the majority of calories and no limit is set as energy requirements can vary significantly from person to person. Good intake of non-starchy vegetables, as these are very low in carbohydrate, is preferred.

3. What are the foods to avoid?

Any food that is high in carbs should be limited

- Grains like rice, wheat, ragi, oats and millet and processed breakfast cereals
- Fruit: most fruits except small portions of berries
- Root vegetables: potatoes, sweet potatoes
- Sugary foods: soda, fruit juice, smoothies, cake, ice cream, chocolates
- Unhealthy fats: processed vegetable oils, margarine
- Sugar-free diet foods: sugar-free candies, sweeteners, desserts

4. What kind of foods am I allowed to eat?

You should base the majority of your meals around these foods:

- Meat: poultry
- Fatty fish: salmon, trout, tuna, and mackerel
- Eggs: free range whole eggs
- Butter and cream: organic
- Cheese: unprocessed cheeses like cheddar, goat, cream, blue, or mozzarella

- Nuts and seeds: almonds, walnuts, flaxseeds, pumpkin seeds, chia seeds
- Avocados: whole avocados or freshly made guacamole
- Healthy oils: extra virgin olive oil, cold pressed coconut or groundnut oil, and avocado oil
- Low carb veggies: green veggies, tomatoes, onions, capsicum

5. How long does it take to get adapted to this diet?

With a low carb diet, your body will need the transition from burning glucose to using your body's fat as fuel. It will take a few days or weeks to get used to it. You may experience some gastrointestinal symptoms of carbohydrate withdrawal at first, but once you become fat-adapted, it will be much easier. How long it takes will depend on how strictly you follow the diet and most importantly the duration of your diabetes.

6. Do I need to count or restrict calories?

No, a low carb-healthy fat diet can be eaten to satiety. The principle is - eat when hungry and stop when full and don't feel deprived. Never eat by the clock.

7. Can I reverse Type 1 diabetes?

If you have type 1 diabetes, your pancreas makes little to no insulin and therefore you need to inject insulin regularly to metabolize glucose. Though there is no cure for Type 1 diabetes as of now, and it cannot be reversed, an LCHF diet can help towards bringing down insulin requirement.

8. I am a diabetic for several years – is this diet suitable for me?

Yes, it is suitable. You will need to make modifications to your routine and get adapted to it. You will see good results if you follow the suggested plan.

9. What is the difference between blood sugar and insulin resistance?

Insulin resistance is when cells in the muscles, fat, and liver don't respond well to insulin and can't use the glucose from the blood for energy. To compensate, the pancreas makes more insulin and over time, the blood sugar levels start increasing and this leads to prediabetes and Type 2 diabetes.

10. Will the diet help with weight loss and will it improve my blood pressure and cholesterol levels?

Yes, these are the main benefits of this diet. There will be a reduced dependence on medication, improvements in insulin sensitivity and cholesterol levels, and lower blood pressure levels, besides others. If you are on medication, you will need to speak to your doctor, who will be able to advise you on what precautions to take to reduce the risk of hypoglycemia occurring.

11. Can fatty liver be reversed?

Since eating too much of carbs increases liver fat storage, a low-carb diet results in reduction of liver and abdominal fat. A very-low-carb diet can decrease insulin resistance and insulin levels. Lower insulin levels allow liver fat to be broken down with improvement in liver function tests. Both 'fructose' which is a sugar that occurs naturally in many fruits, and 'sucrose' which is produced naturally in plants, from which white sugar is refined and crystalized, are metabolized in the liver. A reduction in fructose and sucrose can also reduce fatty liver.

12. What are the other health benefits of this diet?

Early studies have now shown that the diet can have added benefits for a wide variety of different health conditions:

- Heart disease
- Cancer
- Alzheimer's disease
- Epilepsy
- Parkinson's disease
- Polycystic ovary syndrome
- Arthritis
- Allergies
- Migraine
- Infertility

13. Will my cholesterol go up when on an LCHF diet?

The concern that following a high-fat and low-carbohydrate diet will cause a spike in cholesterol levels is certainly valid. However, available literature shows that in a majority of people who are on an LCHF diet, there is a reduction in the bad cholesterol, namely triglycerides, and an increase in the good cholesterol, namely HDL

14. Is this diet dangerous for my heart?

An LCHF diet helps reduce the risk factors for heart disease, such as high blood pressure, high cholesterol, prediabetes or type 2 diabetes, and being overweight or obese.

15. What is the 'keto flu' and how can I avoid it?

Your body has always relied on glucose as its primary source of energy. Therefore, when you cut down or reduce carbohydrates drastically, the body's metabolism has to resort to burning fat for energy. This period of adaptation, which can take up to 15 days, can cause symptoms similar to flu like mild weakness or lack of energy. Changes in bowel habits, leg cramps and bad breath are other symptoms.

This state is temporary and keeping yourself well hydrated and managing your electrolytes should help.

16. Can I practice intermittent fasting on keto?

Yes, you can. It is a very useful tool to boost fat burning.

17. After reaching my health goals or target weight, can I go back eating normally?

Not really, it has to be a lifestyle change to see sustained results. While you can compromise for social events and travel, you need to follow the diet for the most part. LCHF uses food as medicine, and going back to the old diet means you will need to go back to taking your medicines again.

18. Are there some tips & tricks to make it easier?

Although it can be challenging to switch to an LCHF diet, the below measures can make it easier:

- Look at food labels and check the grams of fat, carbs, and fiber to determine how they can fit into your diet
- Plan out your meals in advance
- Many websites, food blogs, apps, and cookbooks also offer recipes and meal ideas that you can use to build your own custom menu
- Some meal delivery services even offer keto-friendly options for a quick and convenient way to enjoy keto meals at home.

- When going to social gatherings or visiting family and friends, you can consider taking your own food, which can make it much easier to limit intake of carbs and stick to your meal plan. You could also have your meal before you leave home. If you are dining in a place where options for LCHF are limited, you can have proteins instead.

19. Is the LCHF diet suitable for all?

The LCHF diet is ideal for those who wish to lose weight, reduce the risk of lifestyle diseases, enhance insulin sensitivity and reverse Type 2 diabetes. It is never too early or never too late to start an LCHF diet. 'The best time to fix the roof is when the sun is shining'.

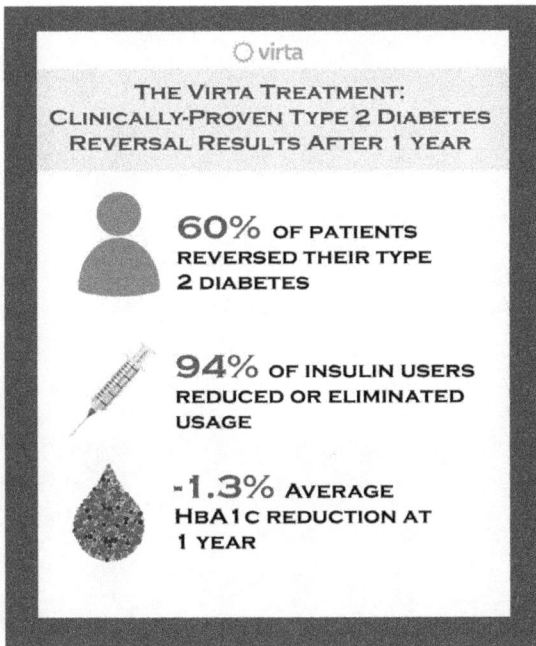

Fig. 34: Benefits of a low carb diet in diabetics (Source: Virta)

PART B:
HAPPINESS AND PEACE

A road to self-discovery

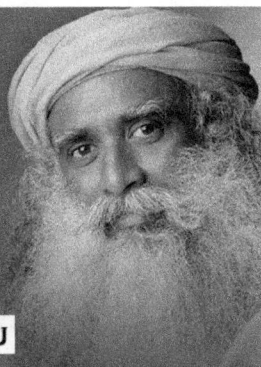

WHAT HAPPENS AROUND
YOU IS NOT ALWAYS
THE WAY YOU WANT.
WHATEVER HAPPENS
WITHIN YOU IS ABSOLUTELY
YOUR MAKING.
THIS IS CALLED KARMA.
IF YOU DO NOT TAKE CHARGE
OF THIS THEN YOU BECOME
AN ACCIDENTAL LIFE.

- SADGURU

Fig 35: We can and must control our inner selves

20

THE OUTER AND INNER SELF

"Mental health is not a destination, but a process.
It's about how you drive, not where you
are going"
— Noam Shpancer

The World Health Organization (WHO) defines "health" as a state of complete physical, mental and social well-being and not merely the absence of disease or infirmity. The definition lends itself to the expansive nature of how health of an individual and a community is both evaluated and protected. While physical health is more tangibly measured and spoken about, mental health gets less respect than it deserves. With mental health, there is another perspective of spiritual health. Often spirituality is confused with religion and rituals. In reality mental and spiritual health are two sides of the same coin. When we foster positive thoughts in our minds and perform actions without an ego, with passion and compassion we welcome peace and happiness in our lives.

A strong mind is the master of a strong body. In the previous section we looked at how the health of our physical bodies is a result of what we eat and metabolize and how that directly and indirectly influences our ability to combat common lifestyle diseases. In this section, we will delve into how we must be aware of and care about our "inner bodies", our mental health, and our spiritual well-being with the aim of achieving sustainable peace and happiness.

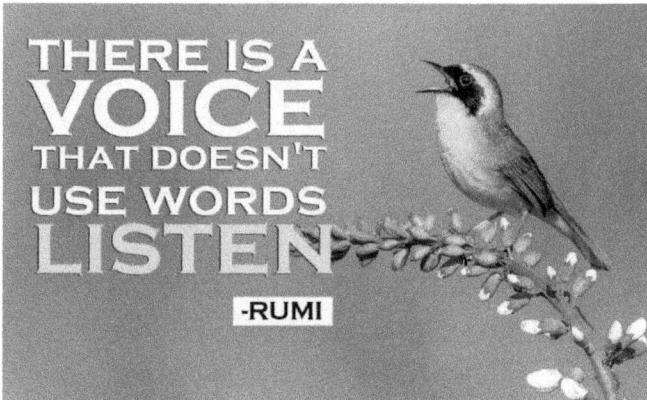

Fig 36: "Our subconscious mind helps us work simultaneously. There are trillions of perfectly coordinated harmonious actions that take place while performing these activities."

Human Body Is the Best Work of Art:

The human body is the most fabulous creation we can ever encounter. Look at the intricate detailing of our organs, and the intelligence that has been programmed into our brains! The numbers are mind-boggling! Can you imagine how our heart beats about 1,00,000 times a day and about 35 million times a year! It pumps six litres of blood through 1,20,000 kilometers of blood vessels in a day—that is equivalent of encircling the Earth two and a half times!

In one second, we produce about 1.2 million red blood cells which are just enough to replace an equal number of cells that die. All this is accomplished with such accuracy and consistency!

The main unit of the human body is cells — an average adult human body contains a whopping 100 trillion cells. Cells are the fundamental units that build our human body. We survive and thrive only because of the work that is efficiently done by every cell in our body. Each cell is designed with a particular purpose and function.

Expensive man-made digital cameras can capture up to 400 megapixels currently. Our eyes on the other hand can view up to 576 megapixels. Furthermore, the human eye can differentiate between thousands of colors. Interestingly, the muscle that controls our eyelids is the fastest muscle in the body. An average person will blink approximately 15,000 times a day.

The digestive system consists of several organs such as the mouth, esophagus, stomach, small intestine, larger intestine, rectum, and anus, which work together to break down and absorb food and remove waste from the body. The liver and pancreas also play a significant role.

Our digestive and metabolic systems also have the remarkable ability to transform the food we eat into energy that is required for the proper functioning of the body. The immune system is like our personal bodyguard. Our body is vulnerable without an immune system and is open to all kinds of bacteria, viruses, and parasites. Our immune system keeps us healthy while we encounter a vast number of pathogens.

Whenever there is a cut on your skin, have you noticed how the wound heals in layers? There is a tremendous amount of activity that happens in and around the wound to seal and heal it. When you think about the level of protection, our body's defense system is more reliable than the security systems that guard the presidents and prime ministers of the greatest of nations.

Living beings can reproduce, due to our reproductive system. Ensuring the survival of our species is its primary role. The way our reproductive system is designed and the mechanism of fertilizing an egg and turning it into a fully-grown baby is beyond our intelligence.

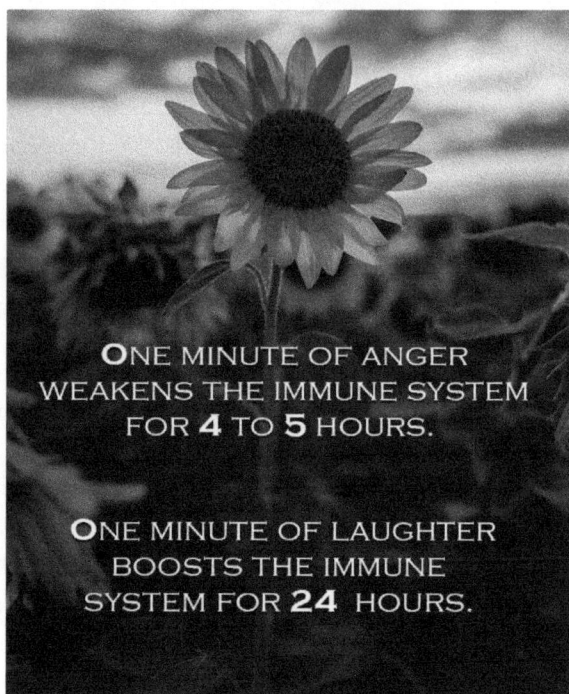

Fig 37: Staying happy boosts our immunity

Our brain is like the Central Processing Unit. It masters the entire body, gives instructions, and controls all our activities, including our feelings, memories, and even the way we perceive information. Yet, at an individual level, we all have limited capabilities.

Imagine you are typing a letter while watching a show on the TV and you suddenly receive a phone call. How well can you perform all three tasks? In reality, our conscious mind can perform only one or two tasks at a time effectively.

On the other hand, our inner intelligence helps us work on several processes simultaneously. Inner intelligence can perform trillions of perfectly coordinated harmonious actions. This clearly shows that there are two sides to each one of us: The outer limited version and the inner unimaginably intelligent and limitless self. Though externally we have different capabilities, internally, all of us are the same with equal capabilities.

Man's Relationship with The Universe:

We humans must aim to become one with our inner intelligence. As long as we identify ourselves with our body, we limit ourselves to our body. But, when we identify ourselves with our spirit, we can harness the unlimited power and intelligence of our spirit. The body and the spirit can be compared to a light bulb and electricity. Here's how: We have several electric appliances that are used for various purposes. However, the one thing that drives all these appliances is electricity. Similarly, we all have different bodies, but the spirit in all of us is the same and drives us all.

Imagine a dog locked in a small room with mirrors on all four walls. On seeing thousands of its own images in the mirror, out of its disillusion and ignorance, the dog barks and bites itself endlessly until it ultimately drops down in exhaustion.

The moral here is that humans will also end up like that dog if we identify ourselves with the body. The moment we realize the truth, everything automatically falls into place, and we find that the thousands of images around us are our own, and we start to smile and embrace them with eternal love. Where there is deep love, words are virtually unnecessary as most of the communication is through feelings - the language of the soul.

Everything and everyone in this universe are connected to the force of life or an infinite energy source. It is one life that manifests in countless forms. All living things on the planet share the same soul and, in this way, all of us are connected to one another.

The tragedy is when the notion of individuality sets in. It is the root cause of all evil. There are two sides to each one of us. First is the outer cover that is different for every individual. The second one is the inner content, which is more intelligent and powerful than the outer cover. This inner content is the same within all of us. So, let us identify with the content and not the cover.

This explanation leads us to the conclusion that life is eternal, and that there is only one of us here. The day we realize this and believe in this theory is when we can stop struggling and start living, and on that day, our need for everything else ends. We can then move through life as if everyone and everything reflects ourselves, and can feel one with everyone. Let us identify with the inner intelligence and not the body.

"There is an intelligence within all of us that digests the food we consume and keeps our heart beating. It created you and me. It knows the way better than any of us."

21

WHY ARE WE IN THE
PRESENT STATE?

"Whether you think you can, or think you can't...
you're right."
— Henry Ford

We are all familiar with the saying 'what you sow, so shall you reap.' It's true, isn't it? If I hurt you, then your most probable reaction would be to hurt me back. If I accuse you, you will blame me. If I love you, you will love me back. If I see good in you, you will see good in me. Over the years, as a physician dealing with patients and their caregivers, I have seen these emotions manifest reciprocally. Most often, we live in our minds. Yet we do not pay attention to what goes on in it – our thoughts. Our circumstances are what we think they are. We create our reality by constantly having thoughts about it until we start believing it to be true.

When we have incessant thoughts about something, it leads us to start believing them as reality. For instance, if we believe that we are not good enough every minute of the day, we will end up striving hard to prove ourselves, not to others, but to ourselves.

On the other hand, when our mind thinks constructive thoughts, we end up being productive. Our positive thoughts and opinions get deposited in our subconscious minds. This part of our mind is magically powerful. It is a storehouse of our personality traits and is built on the wealth of our experiences. It helps us respond to situations. If we are to become people who respond and not react, then we must sow the right ideas in our minds. We must have positive thoughts so that we can reach our destination. Our mind is the link between our body and the subconscious. It is through this instrument that we can influence the subconscious to work for, or against us.

We do not have to change or control anybody or anything outside of us to keep ourselves happy. All we need to do is watch our minds very carefully and slowly acquire control over it to work in our favor. This practice is learned by conscious and deliberated practice. All religious processes like prayers, contemplation, meditation, and more are small ways and means of influencing our inner intelligence through our minds. To control one's mind, we must first quieten it. Remember, an idle mind may be the devil's workshop, but a quiet mind is nature's workplace. If we were to only look around us, we would notice that a vast majority of us live in the world on the outside, whereas the more enlightened men and women are intensely interested in the world within.

We must remember that it is the world within our thoughts and feelings that make the world outside of us. If we want to have better surroundings, we must get to the cause, and this cause is within us, i.e., our thoughts and beliefs. Change them, and the outer world will change automatically. Our subconscious mind is susceptible to our ideas. Our life is the way it is because of the choices we make or fail to make.

Observe a person who complains all the time and is happy with nothing in his or her life. You will notice that their entire life is filled with misfortunes. On the other hand, a happy-go-lucky, humorous, joyous person attracts only happiness throughout their lives. Notice another person whom you envy. It may seem that he or she has everything you could wish for—an ideal spouse, loving children, plenty of money, lots of free time, fame and power, and popularity.

If you notice their attitude, you will see that they are delightful people, who accept what comes their way, never complaining or condemning anybody, and never desperate for anything. All good things seem to follow them.

Now that we are done with our little observation, let us work to change our attitudes for our benefit. But first, we must not only learn how things work, but we must believe in them as well. If we have even an iota of doubt, or if we make half-hearted attempts, or if we do not have the patience to wait for the results, then things will not work out for us. Faith is everything. Believe that you deserve it and that you can achieve it.

To further exercise control over our thoughts, we must first learn to watch and observe them. We must try to see what is going on within us. Observe how our minds can never stay on one subject for a long time? The more our mind runs untethered, the fickler it becomes. We must learn to control these thoughts and tame them.

Once we practice this, only then will we be able to observe and distinguish between necessary and unnecessary thoughts. All sorts of thoughts run through our minds—good, bad, and ugly. Since nobody else has access to our minds, do we have the liberty to think numerous things about several people? This is actually where we go wrong. If we consistently think bad about a particular person, then these thoughts automatically attract a similar response from that person and before you know it, your thoughts manifest in your actions. People around us behave just the way we expect them to act towards us.

Our belief in ourselves and positivity are crucial for our minds. The greatest battles are won and lost in the mind. So, picture yourself winning, always.

22

WATCHING OUR THOUGHTS

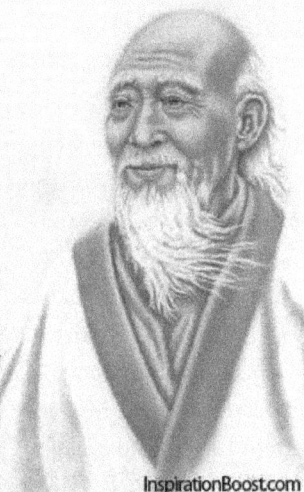

> Watch your thoughts;
>   They become words.
> Watch your words;
>   They become actions.
> Watch your actions;
>   They become habits.
> Watch your habits;
>   They become character.
> Watch your character;
>   It becomes your destiny.
>
> **Lao Tzu**
>
> InspirationBoost.com

Fig 38: You become what you think you are

Ralph Waldo Emerson, one of the greatest philosophers of our time, had once said, 'A man is what he thinks all day long.' Simply put, our thoughts and actions define us. Thoughts, like breathing, can either be deliberate or automatic. Just as we can breathe deliberately, we can choose to think about a specific problem or situation. Conscious thinking is one of the gifts of being human. But when the mind isn't focused, unwanted thoughts come up. It is rather unfortunate that we have to juggle our way through so much clutter.

The human mind is usually compared to a monkey—always restless, wandering, never idle. To exercise control over our thoughts, we must first learn to watch and observe them. We must try to see what is going on within us. Observe how our minds can never stay on one subject for a long time. The more our mind runs untethered, the fickler it becomes. You have to know this. All our thoughts need not be just stories. They can be a series of things - past events, present situations, or future plans. We must learn to control these thoughts and tame them.

Once we practice this, then we can start analyzing what is happening in our minds. We can soon be able to observe and distinguish between the necessary thoughts and get rid of the unnecessary thoughts.

Since we feel confident that nobody else has access to our minds, we take the liberty of thinking numerous thoughts about several people. This is where we go wrong. If we consistently think wrongly of a particular person, then these thoughts automatically attract a similar response from that very person, and the reverse also is true.

Also, before you know it, your thoughts show up in the way you act. People around us behave just the way we expect them to act with us. Our spouses, children, superiors, helpers, and the whole world respond to our expectations. Have you noticed that when we expect our children to be responsible, they live up to it? When we expect them to be irresponsible, they do exactly so. You might have noticed that all your subordinates behave in the same manner, for the way they behave has nothing to do with them; it has everything to do with you.

So, even though we may get to know new people, their behaviour will be similar to the old ones because the common factor is us. If we expect a person to be rude and demanding, then that is what he will be, and if we hope and believe him to be loving, caring and working for our benefit, then that is how he will respond to us.

However, specific thoughts tend to stick with us. It is often the thoughts with a powerful emotional pull that we have difficulty in letting go of. It is like our emotions having a strong bonding that make us think of something particularly, where they remain stuck and however hard we try, they just don't go away. We can't easily let go of our thoughts often. Here's what I suggest. Close your eyes and visualize these thoughts like passing clouds. Don't hold on to them. Just observe them and let them float away. I am reminded of a story I read about how our thoughts can be manipulated by our external environment.

Once there was a man. He lived in one of the most beautiful houses in the town with his three sons. The man loved his house a lot! Though many had offered to buy it for double the price, he had never agreed to sell it. The man usually had to travel outside his town on work. Once, when he came back from work, he found that his house was on fire. Though hundreds of people had gathered, no one could do anything and it was just burning before his eyes. The fire had spread so far that even if it was put out, nothing could be saved. This made the man very sad.

The man's eldest son came running up to him and whispered in his ear: "Don't be worried father. I sold the house yesterday and at a very good price - three times the usual price. The offer was so good I could not wait for you. Forgive me." The man said, "Thank God, this house is not ours now!" Then he relaxed and became a silent spectator, just like the others.

Please think about it! Just a moment before, the man was not an observer, and was attached to the house. Though everything - the house and the fire - were the same, after talking to his son, the man became unattached. In fact, he started enjoying the spectacle, just like everybody else in the crowd.

Then the man's second son came running to him and said, "What are you doing father? Why are you smiling when the house is on fire?" The man said, "Don't you know, your brother has sold the house." The son said, "Yes, but we have only received the advance, not the entire amount. I doubt now that the buyer is going to purchase it."

Again, the situation changes!! The tears which had disappeared came back to the man's eyes. He lost his smile and his heart started beating faster. The 'watcher' was gone. He was once again attached to the house.

Then the third son came and told him, "Father, the buyer is a man of his word. I have just spoken to him and he told me that it doesn't matter whether the house is on fire or not, he will pay us the price that we had settled on as neither us nor him knew that the house would catch fire."

Once again the joy was back and the family became 'watchers'! The attachment was no longer there. Actually nothing was changing but the feeling of ownership towards the house, which made all the difference.

So, what is the moral here? We are as attached to something as our mind wants us to believe.

"We can't prevent crows from flying over our heads, but we can certainly prevent them from putting their nests up there."

23

WE ARE ACTORS ALL DAY LONG!

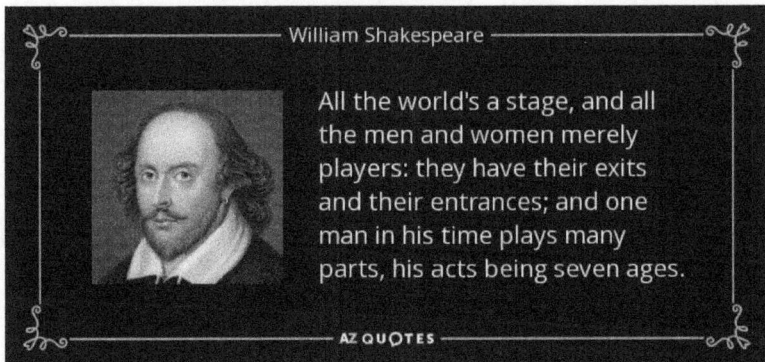

> William Shakespeare
>
> All the world's a stage, and all the men and women merely players: they have their exits and their entrances; and one man in his time plays many parts, his acts being seven ages.
>
> AZ QUOTES

Fig. 39: In playing our different roles in life, let us now forget who we really are

If this isn't the truest thing that has been said, I don't know what is. This quote resonates with me at a deeper level. Let me explain. As our day begins, we are up and ready to face the world and do what needs to be done.

We take up responsibilities and play different roles during the day. At first, we're soldiers facing the daily grind. We are spouses, parents at the breakfast table, and strong-headed bosses in the office cabins. As the sun sets, we are friends in coffee shops who laugh at silly jokes or loving parents or grandparents playing with the kids. Take a moment here. Did you notice that we all play different roles in different situations? We switch roles based on the demands of the situation we face. However, in imbibing all the traits that are expected of us in our different performances, we tend to forget who we actually are and what our real self is! We often do not reveal our true selves to anyone, and this process is involuntary. We unknowingly become a part of the world, and at some point, we lose track of our own identity.

I strongly believe that in every part of the day, we should be aware of the difference between the 'role' we are playing and the 'real' person behind it. We must never forget that we are merely playing a character just as others are playing their roles in life's ever-unfolding drama. I was once witnessing a film shooting. It was a fight scene wherein the hero beats up the villain. After the scene was completed, I was surprised to see the hero walk up to the villain, touch his feet, and ask for forgiveness. The person playing the villain was a senior artist and an elderly man and the hero, out of respect, made sure he apologized to him.

In real life, we may not be able to physically touch the feet of those we wrong and say 'sorry'. Here's a tip. Ask for forgiveness mentally from all the people you might have wronged. Also, every time you are with someone, act like it is your last day with them and see how your behavior changes. When we realize that everyone is an extension of ourselves, our behavior towards them automatically changes.

For example, if we suddenly bump into an Indian in a foreign country, we tend to stop and start a conversation. We are strangers, yet there's some kind of connection. Similarly, if we recognize and accept that everyone is but an extension of ourselves, the forces of nature will begin to work in our favor.

Acceptance of each other is vital to maintain peace, justice, and harmony not just in the world around us, but in the world within.

Asking for forgiveness does not make anyone weak. In fact, it is an act of grace and bravery. It takes a lot of courage to be able to accept one's mistakes and right a wrong. Don't forget to forgive the people who have hurt you.

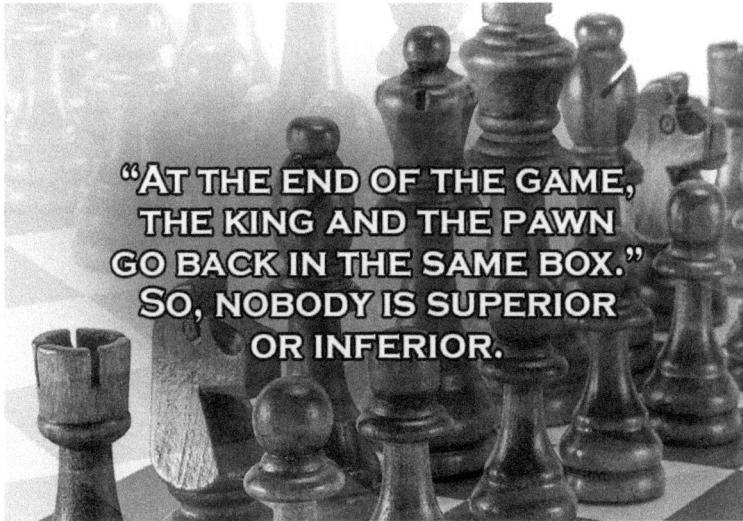

Fig 40: Our designations are not our true self

Forgive them not because they deserve forgiveness but because you deserve peace. A quick checklist to successful relationships is to remind ourselves that we play 'roles' all day. Our designation is not our personality or identity. Everyone has a facade. We must know our true selves by being self-aware. If we treat everyone equally and with basic dignity, our relationships will be strong. It is important to forgive and also seek forgiveness when we are wrong.

24

REACTION VS RESPONSE

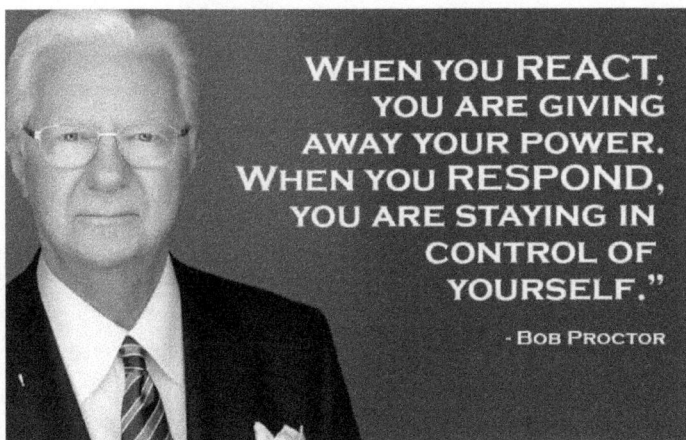

Fig 41: A response combines the maturity of the conscious and the subconscious mind

Reaction versus response is my favorite topic. It is the predicament that I like to indulge in because it gives me a sense of control. It also allows me to be a better version of myself.

Let me ask you this. What do you do when someone says something mean to you? What is your first reaction?

Do you feel bad and take whatever the person said to heart and feel sorry for yourself? Or, do you 'give it back' in the same measure or more? Simply put, do you react, or do you respond? Do you reply negatively or positively? Are you comfortable with the result of the whole encounter? If these questions are on your mind after every argument, then continue reading further.

Before we begin, let us understand what it means to 'react' and to 'respond'. A reaction is often a defense mechanism. It is an immediate, 'knee jerk' action and more often than not something you may regret later. A response, on the other hand, usually occurs more slowly. It is based on information from both the conscious mind and the subconscious mind.

With respect to arguments, one needs to understand that one can either react or respond to a concept or an idea that is put forth. When one is reacting, the subconscious mind is the major player. It is providing inputs derived from one's subconscious mind, which is pre-programmed. It is driven by nature, therefore, also impulsive and automatic. In such a situation, we have very little control.

Indeed, the situation is controlling us. For instance, you are driving to work, and there is a minor disagreement with someone on the road. You can either be calm and sort out the differences amicably or have a fight and create a scene on the street. In the first scenario, the problem is sorted out, and there are no hard feelings. In the second situation, someone is bound to get hurt.

Now, as people, when things get tricky, we must think about the consequences before acting out. Since we were kids, we have been trained to be good to good people and bad to bad people. We believe it is natural to pay people back with the same coin. Is it honestly possible to be good to the person who is bad to you?

To answer this question, we need to take a step back and weigh our options. How else can we respond to people that hurt us or make us angry?

Our options are to be:

1) rude to them,
2) ignore them, or
3) give them the benefit of the doubt.

When you think about a particular interaction with another person, if you have impulsively said whatever comes to your mind, then you are merely reacting. But if you choose from any of the aforementioned options after some thought, then you are responding. You are doing better. You are treating the other person better than they have treated you. Is this fair? Is it possible to kiss the feet that kick us?

Yes. Why not! Don't we do the same thing with babies? We know that babies are innocent, and we love them. So, my question is, if we can be patient with babies, then why not with everyone else? Why can't we give them the benefit of the doubt and let things go? Have mercy and forgive people.

Always assume the best about people. Because when you think good, it is easier to do better. The key is to understand that our inner-state needs to reflect our outer conditions and vice versa. For instance, if you are calm and confident, then no matter how stressful the situation is, you will remain composed. If you can be positive in a negative situation – you win!

I came across this long ago in the "Speaking Tree" column of Times of India. This is worth a read. "Millions of people are suffering undeserved stress, trials, problems, and heartache. They never seem to be a success in life. Bad days follow bad days. Terrible things seem to be constantly happening. There's constant stress, lack of joy, and broken relationships. Worry consumes time, anger breaks friendships, and life seems dreary and is not enjoyed to the fullest. Friends are lost. Life is a bore and often seems cruel." Does this describe you? If so, do not be discouraged. You can be different!

Understand and apply the 90/10 secret. It will change your life! Ten percent of life is made up of what happens to you. Ninety percent of life is decided by how you react.

What does this mean? We really have no control over ten percent of what happens to us. We cannot stop the car from breaking down. The plane may arrive late, which throws our whole schedule off. A driver may cut us off in traffic. We have no control over this 10 percent. The other 90 percent is different. You determine the other 90 percent! How? By your reaction.

You cannot control a red light, but you can control your reaction.

Let's use an example - You're eating breakfast with your family. Your daughter knocks over a cup of coffee onto your business shirt. You have no control over what just happened. What happens next will be determined by how you react. You curse. You harshly scold your daughter for knocking the coffee cup over. She breaks down in tears.

After scolding her, you turn to your spouse and criticize her for placing the cup too close to the edge of the table. A short verbal battle follows. You storm upstairs and change your shirt. Back downstairs you find your daughter has been too busy crying to finish breakfast and get ready for school. She misses the bus. Your spouse must leave immediately for work. You rush to the car and drive your daughter to school. Because you are late, you drive 60 km per hour in a 45-kmph speed limit. You still get delayed and you arrive at school, 15 minutes late. Your daughter runs to the building without saying goodbye.

After arriving at the office 20 minutes late, you find you forgot your briefcase. Your day has started badly. As it continues, it seems to get worse and worse. You look forward to going home. When you arrive home, you find a small wedge in your relationship with your spouse and daughter. Why? Because of how you reacted in the morning. Why did you have a bad day? You had no control over what happened with the coffee. How you reacted in those five seconds is what caused your bad day.

Here is what could have and should have happened. Coffee

splashes over you. Your daughter is about to cry. You gently say "It's OK honey, you just need to be more careful next time". Grabbing a towel, you rush upstairs.

After grabbing a new shirt and your briefcase, you come back down in time to look through the window and see your child getting on the school bus. She turns and waves. You reach your office five minutes early and cheerfully greet the staff. Your boss comments on how good a day you are having. Notice the difference? Two different scenarios. Both started the same. Both ended differently. Why? Because of how you "REACTED". Here are some ways to apply the 90/10 secret. If someone says something negative about you, do not be a sponge.

Let the attack roll off like water on glass. React properly and it will not ruin your day. A wrong reaction could result in you losing a friend, getting stressed out, etc. How do you react if someone cuts you off in traffic? Do you lose your temper? Pound the steering wheel? Do you curse? Does your blood pressure skyrocket? Do you try and bump them? WHO CARES if you arrive ten minutes late to work? Why let the blue car ruin your drive? Remember the 90-10 principle, and do not worry about it! You are told you lost your job. Why lose sleep or get irritated? It will work out. Use your "worrying" energy into finding another job.

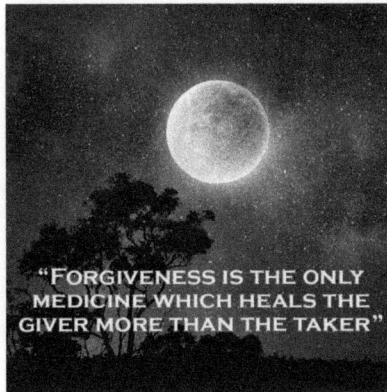

Fig 42: Stay compassionate and be quick to forgive

#

To give another example, the plane is late and it is going to upset your schedule for the day. Why take out your frustration on the flight attendant? She has no control over what is going on. Use your time to study, or get to know the other passengers. Why get stressed out? It will just make things worse.

You now know the 90/10 secret. Apply it and you will be amazed at the results. To make the best of any situation, keep telling yourself three things,

1) it doesn't really matter,
2) it is ok,
3) so what?

The bigger picture is what matters. Always appreciate your problems, it makes you stronger. We must learn to focus on the solution, and not on the problem!

"Every time you are tempted to react in the same old way, ask if you want to be a prisoner of the past or a pioneer of the future."
— Deepak Chopra

25

BELIEF VS TRUTH

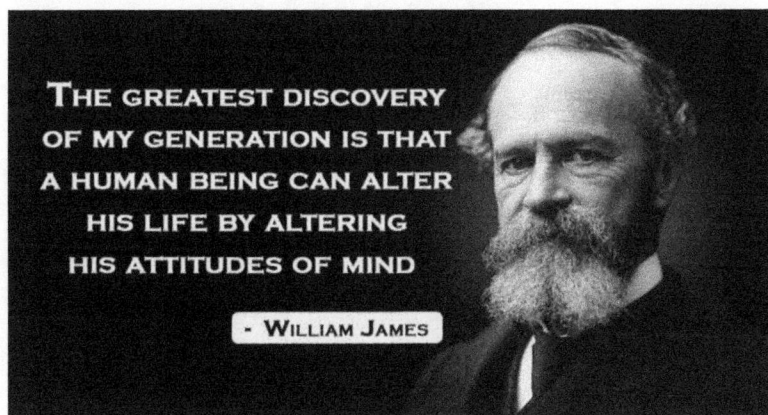

THE GREATEST DISCOVERY
OF MY GENERATION IS THAT
A HUMAN BEING CAN ALTER
HIS LIFE BY ALTERING
HIS ATTITUDES OF MIND

- WILLIAM JAMES

Fig 43: Our thoughts form the person we are

I like to believe that our relationships are built on our words and actions towards one another. The truth, however, is that our relationships are based on what we think about others.

Our thoughts are compelling and have a bearing on us more than we would like them to. If we are under the assumption that thoughts do not hurt others, we are wrong. For instance, if we have negative thoughts about someone, they will turn into actions in no time. Our thoughts *form* the person we are. "As the thought so the man." If we think and behave well today, we will be happy tomorrow. If we are not happy as we are, where we are, how we are, here and now, we will never be satisfied tomorrow or the day after. We have this misconception that we will be happy when we get there, or when we acquire a particular thing. But the truth is, if we are happy as we are, we will acquire whatever we want more easily, simply because we are in a better mindset to work towards it and achieve it.

We also believe that if we are hungry for more, we will achieve and get more. The truth is, if we desire things that are out of our reach, irrespective of what we achieve, we will always be left wanting for more. There will be no end to our desires. We believe that we are stressed out by people and circumstances, but the truth is that people or situations do not cause stress. It is our *reactions* to these various circumstances that generate stress. Our responses and reactions are in our control. As the driver of your life, you should know better! We believe that we need to fight a hundred battles every day, but the truth is that we need to fight only one battle – the one between us and our minds. This is an important battle which decides whether we win or lose in this game called 'life'.

To be happy, we need to do only one thing, and that is to keep our minds happy. We can do this easily by training the mind to look at the silver lining behind every cloud. Whatever be the situation, focus on the good parts of it. Don't bother whether the glass is half full or half empty. Be happy that you have a glass and something in it. Don't sit around waiting for things to get more comfortable, simpler, and better. They never will. Life will always be complicated. So, learn to be happy right now; otherwise, you will run out of time. God forbid you have an accident and lose an eye; you should be thankful that you didn't lose both your eyes. If you did lose both your eyes, then be grateful that you are alive.

Give people the benefit of doubt. Remember, everyone you come across in your life is dealing with a battle of their own. So, try to be kind. Live by the principle of accepting and respecting all. So, instead of complaining about the circumstances or people you have to deal with, start by asking the following questions:

1) Do I have to respond to all?

2) Can I give the benefit of the doubt and forgive?

3) Will it really matter in the long run?

Make sure that your response passes the above test, and you are good to go. While you are at it, remember that the easiest way to receive anything is just to wish it for others. What goes around comes around. We are often under the assumption that our journey affects our state of mind. However, in reality, it is the other way round. It is your state of mind that affects the journey. You can fix this by learning to dissociate the external conditions from your inner reaction. Whenever there is an unpleasant situation, the mind goes into overdrive. The easiest way to neutralize the mind is to accept the situation you are in. If you can't change the situation, then simply surrender to it— being stuck in a traffic jam, for instance. If you go a little deeper into this argument, you will realize that everybody and every situation is a part of your journey. Do not see things as obstacles, rather see them as a part of your 'Karmic Journey.'

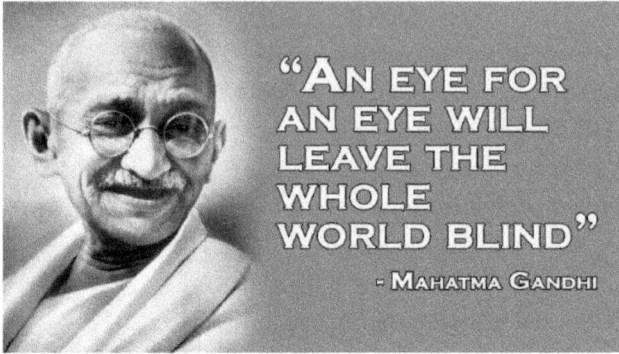

Fig 44: Be kind. Respect and Accept all

Don't blame any circumstance, or resent anyone. Accept everything and learn to take responsibility for it. This will remove or at least reduce your suffering in any situation. Ultimately, you need to ask yourself this: Why worry about things that are not in your control? If the mind doesn't see it as a problem, then it's not a problem, as simple as that. Give people the benefit of the doubt. Remember, everyone you come across in your life is dealing with a battle of their own. Be like a thermostat and not a thermometer. A thermometer keeps changing with the environment, whereas a thermostat changes the environment. Don't blame a situation or a person. Accept your fate and learn to take responsibility for it.

"The world says you must have it all to be happy, but the soul says be happy and you shall have it all."

26

"In your soul are infinitely precious things that cannot be taken from you."
-Oscar Wilde

RELATIONSHIP BETWEEN ROLE AND SOUL

The ultimate aim of all human beings is to be happy and live in peace. As people, we have been chasing this utopia all our lives. We have looked for solutions across borders from different countries and customs, yet it remains elusive. The ultimate truth is, if you want to be happy, you need to see everyone as an extension of yourself. It is similar to a dog looking at its own image in the mirror and is unable to recognize it.

Likewise, each of us is unable to recognize the other person as an extension of ourselves due to our ignorance. We judge people only by the cover -- the body, the status, and the name. But in reality, it's only the cover that is different. If you can go a little deeper, you will find that the contents in each of us is one and the same.

As I mentioned in the previous chapters, there is this energy of 'life', 'soul' or 'spirit' whatever you may choose to call it. It is that intelligence that converts what we eat and drink into flesh and blood. It is that power that built this body, and every organ, while also ensuring its function. We must realize that, while we may be playing different roles during the day, at the end of our journey, the pawn and the king go into the same box. Therefore, we must have regard for the roles but we must not take them too seriously. Likewise, all people are alike because everyone has the same soul. So, we must respect and care for everyone equally. Let us consider this analogy; in a play, one may be a king and the other a servant. This is only a role that lasts as long as you are on the stage. After the play is over, the king is neither superior nor is the servant inferior. They are both equal. The problem is that we take our roles too seriously and create the construct of superior and inferior in our minds.

Let us assume you are going to meet the prime minister. As you get into the car, you order the driver to take you to the PM's house. On the way, if he is not driving correctly, you admonish him. At the security, you behave differently with the guards. At the reception you are courteous, and confident when you meet the PM's secretary. However, when you meet the PM, you are humble and extremely respectful. Basically, you are a different person every time depending upon the status of the individual you have interacted with. There can be little doubt that external courtesy can be based upon the position but the true 'respect' you ought to give to another human being has to be the same no matter who you are dealing with. Respect should never change based on the role. Because ideally, respect is for the soul and it should be the same for everyone. Besides being respectful, we must be kind.

Compassion Is Key

No matter what, we must remember that we are humans. And human beings make mistakes. We are flawed. So, when someone makes a mistake, instead of becoming judgemental, hurt or angry, we need to be compassionate. We must strive to understand their insecurity or ignorance that made them commit an error. We all fail at times. The person who wronged you may be going through tough times. They could be in pain. We may not agree with them, but we can be kind. That is the essence of treating others as you would like them to treat you. For we are not perfect, we also make mistakes and we would also like to be forgiven.

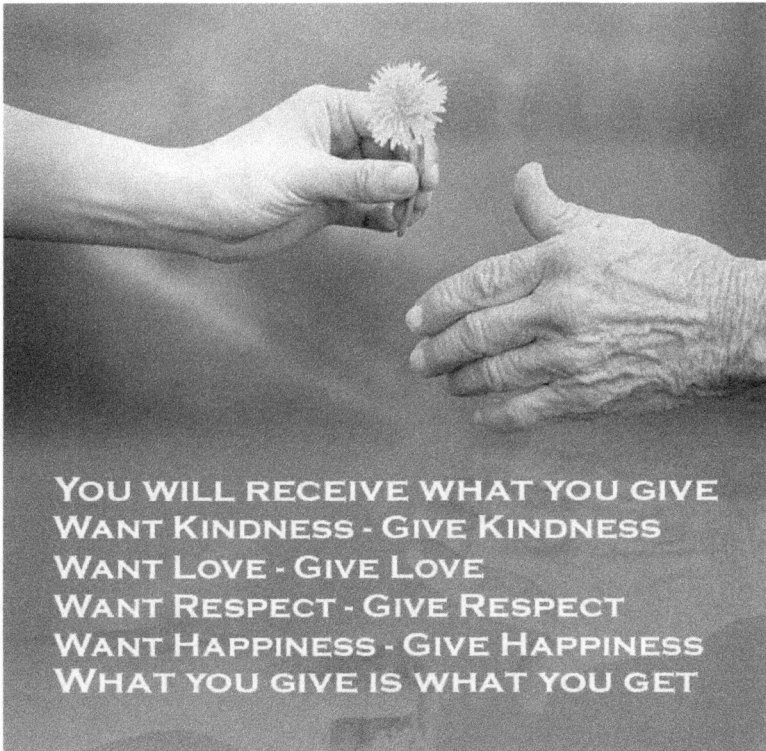

Fig 45: *The best way to get something is to wish it for others. What goes around, comes around!*

27

"Believe in your infinite potential.
Your only limitations are those you set upon yourself."
— *Roy T. Bennett*

IN TUNE WITH YOUR CHEMICALS

Most of us are familiar with the concept of 'hormones'. These are chemical messengers that are secreted by special glands in our bodies and are a means by which our body communicates with itself. In a larger sense, these messengers are responsible for the way our mind and body work together.

Although the more well-known hormones are thyroid hormone, pituitary hormones, estrogen, progesterone and testosterone, there are lesser-known ones as well that play an important role in how we feel, behave and live. In fact, much of our behaviour towards one another is directed and modulated by these hormones. The four hormones that promote happiness are dopamine, oxytocin, serotonin and endorphin. Instead of waiting for these hormones to

143

be secreted, certain actions we may do, or our thoughts have the power of producing these 'happiness' hormones.

Dopamine is called the 'reward' hormone and as the name suggests, it is triggered by praise, a victory, an accomplishment and even food. Sometimes making small 'to-dos' lists and accomplishing them one by one, will give you a dopamine rush. You don't have to wait to achieve that one big landmark! Eating your favourite food and listening to your favourite music also help in dopamine release.

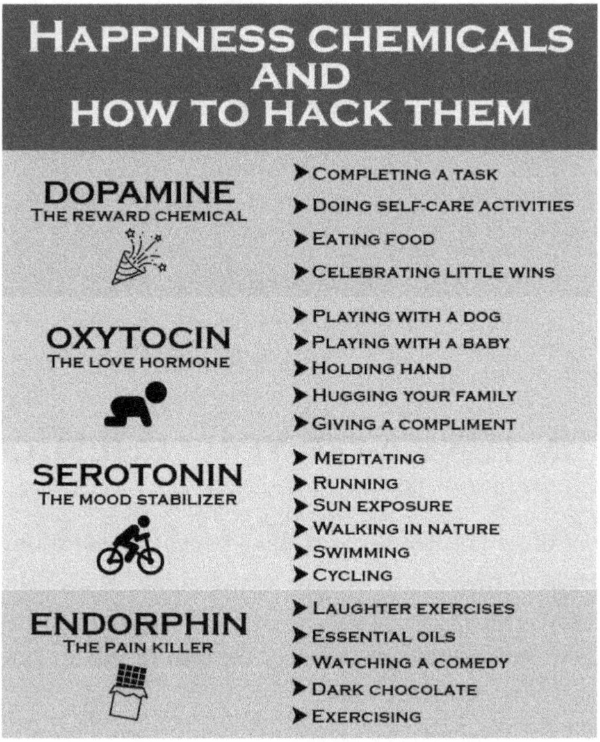

HAPPINESS CHEMICALS AND HOW TO HACK THEM

DOPAMINE
THE REWARD CHEMICAL
- COMPLETING A TASK
- DOING SELF-CARE ACTIVITIES
- EATING FOOD
- CELEBRATING LITTLE WINS

OXYTOCIN
THE LOVE HORMONE
- PLAYING WITH A DOG
- PLAYING WITH A BABY
- HOLDING HAND
- HUGGING YOUR FAMILY
- GIVING A COMPLIMENT

SEROTONIN
THE MOOD STABILIZER
- MEDITATING
- RUNNING
- SUN EXPOSURE
- WALKING IN NATURE
- SWIMMING
- CYCLING

ENDORPHIN
THE PAIN KILLER
- LAUGHTER EXERCISES
- ESSENTIAL OILS
- WATCHING A COMEDY
- DARK CHOCOLATE
- EXERCISING

Fig 46: Our body is a chemical factory of happiness!

Oxytocin is known as the 'bonding hormone'. It is released when we feel safe in the company of those we trust. It has a major role in pregnancy, but outside of that it performs the role of bonding between parents and a child, partners, family units and so on. Simple acts like snuggling, hugging, holding hands, and sharing food, for example, help to secrete oxytocin.

Serotonin is the hormone related to mood regulation. In fact, if it is deficient or inactive, it can lead to clinical depression and psychiatrists use this fact to prescribe medications that can modify the level of serotonin in our brain. The hormone also helps in improving sleep pattern and reducing anxiety. Running, swimming, aerobic exercises, and sunlight improve serotonin levels. Some exercises increase tryptophan, a precursor of serotonin and help in its modulation.

Endorphin is the hormone that is regarded as a natural pain killer. The hormone acts on the same receptors in the brain as very strong pain killers like morphine! It naturally reduces pain, relieves anxiety, and increases pleasure. Exercising, watching a comedy, laughing, dark chocolate, and aromatic oils trigger endorphins.

In conclusion, we have a factory of chemicals in our mind and body that can be conditioned to help us feel better, happy, loved and peaceful. Simple tasks will help in regulating not only a healthy body, but also a peaceful mind.

28

"It's a funny thing about life, once you begin to take note of the things you are grateful for, you begin to lose sight of the things that you lack."
— Germany Kent

THE BOTTOM LINE

Start the day with gratefulness. Be grateful for the things that are of absolute importance to life. What are they? Read on.

Only a drowning man knows the importance of the next breath of air. We will all be gone in a couple of minutes if we don't get our next breath. How grateful are we for that breath of air? We don't even acknowledge it. Try going one day without a drop of water. You can't even imagine it, right? If there is no water, there is literally no life. 70% of our body consists of water, so be grateful for every sip of water you drink.

Scientists have been on a quest to find another planet like Earth for a long time now. No luck as yet. Mother Earth has been supporting all kinds of life forms for billions of years. Thus, humans need to be forever grateful to be living on this planet.

The Sun is the source of light and energy no wonder our ancestors worshipped the Sun. The Sun keeps us warm on a winter's day, provides us with vitamin D, which is very essential for healthy living, and also helps plants in the process of photosynthesis.

Although space is the fifth element, it is as important as all the other four elements that play around it. Space is not just the area around you; the whole cosmos is held in place by this space, without any strings attached! So, bow down before it every morning and evening. We need to appreciate all these elements and thank them every day. Unfortunately, we have got our priorities wrong. We cry over insignificant things and overlook the most essential ones. We constantly prioritize money and luxury over basic things like health, love, peace, joy, freedom, and food. Our minds are too busy finding faults, criticizing, complaining, competing, and controlling. We should stop judging, defending, arguing, and blaming, and avoid resisting, reacting, and resenting, and find time to appreciate all the good things in our lives. The mind always likes to chew on lust, anger, failure, and other hurdles.

Resistance is pain, but acceptance is peace. In any situation, do whatever is possible from the state of acceptance. If nothing can be done, then just surrender. This will keep you stable and at peace. Take responsibility for every situation. Whatever is happening in your life right now, you are responsible for it. At some level, you have attracted them all. Don't blame others for the situation you are in. The more positive you are, the more positivity you will attract. If you see good in others, you will attract better people in your life. Live in the present. Dwelling on a past event does no good to anyone. You are just experiencing the same pain and suffering again and again. On the other hand, by being anxious about the future, you are trying to fight an imaginary thing that may never happen. So, the best thing is to live in the present.

Always pay attention to your inner self and fix that first. All the outer elements will automatically fall into place. What really matters in a pencil is not its wooden cover but the graphite inside. So always pay attention to what is happening inside of you. Sit alone quietly with your eyes closed and introspect regularly. Introspect on the unimaginable intelligence in you that created this body. Reflect on that power that can convert a banana that you have eaten a few hours ago into flesh and blood. Do this every day and notice the vast interconnectedness of life. Have a soul-to-soul relationship, not a role-to-role relationship. Only then can you see the whole Universe as one. If you see all living beings as one, then there will be no criticizing each other, because by doing so, you will be criticizing yourself. 99% of people lead their lives unconsciously, by a force of habit with ingrained traits. The primary reality is inside and the secondary reality is on the outside. Stay compassionate and be quick to forgive. That said, making everyone happy is not in our hands but being happy with everyone is definitely in our hands. Remember this: Gratitude is the healthiest of all human emotions. The more thankful you are, the more things you will have to be thankful for.

The relationship between richness and poverty is similar to the relationship between infinity and zero. It all depends on the scale of comparison with your wants. If your income is more than your desires, you are rich. If your desires are more than your earnings, you are poor. We can consider ourselves rich by reducing our wants. We can become rich not by acquiring lots of money, but by progressively reducing our desires. The problem is not a lack of knowledge but the lack of application. One single step is more significant than all the knowledge in the world. Now, in conclusion, I would like to make one final point – 'Positive Thinking.' Irrespective of the situation, make sure to be determined and have faith in the fact that all things will fall into place eventually. Being anxious about the future is more like fighting a ghost, whose existence you are not even sure of. You are worrying about things that might never happen. Being anxious is also more like tinkering with the mirror because you don't like the image you see in it.

Well, if you want to change the image, you need to change yourself. Sit alone quietly with your eyes closed and introspect.

Reflect on the power that has created you and me.

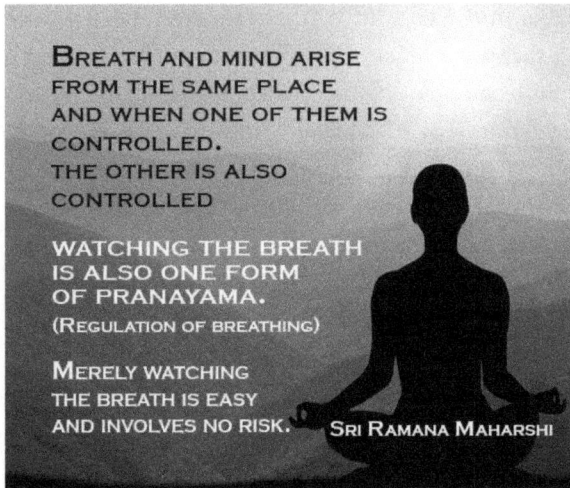

Fig 47: Put life into your years rather than years into your life!

One Story, Two Perspectives

A famous book writer sat in his study. He took out his pen and began to write:

"Last year, I had surgery to remove gallstones. I was bedridden for a long time. In the same year, I turned 60 and was retired ... quitting a company that I loved so much.

I had to leave the job I had been doing for 35 years. That same year I was abandoned by my beloved mother who passed away. Then, still in the same year, my son failed his final medical exam because of a car accident.

Repair costs from the car damage marked the peak of bad luck last year." At the end he wrote: "What a bad year!"

The writer's wife entered the room and found her husband who was sad and pensive. From behind, the wife saw the husband's writing. Slowly she backed away and left the room. fifteen minutes later she came back in and put down a piece of paper with the following words: "Last year, my husband finally managed to get rid of his gallbladder which had been making his stomach hurt for years.

That same year, I am grateful that my husband was able to retire in a healthy and happy state of mind & body. I thank God he was given the opportunity to work and earn for 35 years to support our family. Now, my husband can spend more of his time writing, which has always been his hobby.

In the same year, my 95-year-old mother-in-law, without any pain, returned to God in peace. And still in the same year, God protected our son from harm in a terrible car accident. Our car was seriously damaged by the accident, but my son survived without any serious injuries."

In the last sentence his wife wrote:

"Last year was a year full of extraordinary blessings from God, and we spent it full of wonder and gratitude."

The writer smiled with emotion, and warm tears flowed down his cheeks. He was grateful to his wife for providing him with a different point of view for every incident that he had gone through the past year. A change in his perspective made him appreciate the same events joyfully.

Friends, in this life we must understand that it is not happiness or joy that makes us grateful. It is gratitude that makes us happy/joyful! Let's practice seeing events from a positive point of view and keep envy away from our hearts.

"We can complain because rose bushes have thorns, or rejoice because thorn bushes have roses."
- Abraham Lincoln

29

CONCLUSION

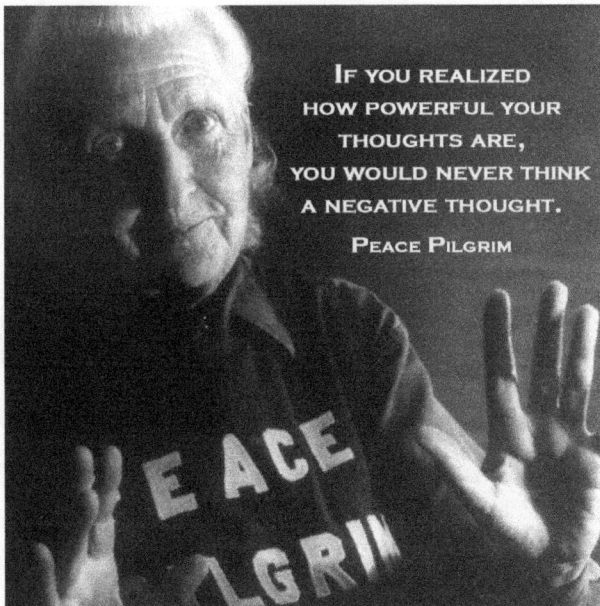

Fig 48: If you realized how powerful your thoughts are, you would never think a negative thought

Humans often judge each other based on their looks, status, and name. It is only the cover that is different. Let us remind ourselves that while we may be playing different roles, at the end of the day, we all belong under the same roof. All of us have the same soul. So, we must respect and care for everyone equally. No one is superior and no one is inferior. We should never take our roles seriously, for it is just a matter of time before we all get off the stage of life.

No matter what, we must remember that we are all humans and human beings make mistakes. We are all flawed. So, when someone makes a mistake, instead of becoming judgmental, hurt, or angry, we need to be compassionate. The person who wronged you may be going through tough times. They could be in pain. We may not agree with them but we can be kind. No one is perfect. Humans are programmed to err; that's how we learn. Treat others as you would like them to treat you.

I have some final thoughts to share with you. Yes, it has to do with spirituality. It doesn't matter if we believe in organized religion or not. We can all agree that there is a power that exists within us. We may not know much about it, but we feel it. We may call it the Universe/Nature/Spirit, and so on. When we are in tune with the infinite, things start to happen instinctively, without any effort. They just fall into place, magically. We suddenly find that we have the time to do all the things we ever wanted to do. We seem to have the necessary money and all the love we require. We tend to move around with a certain glow—the glow of the divine.

We love everyone and everything, and in turn, everyone loves us. We spontaneously fulfill all our needs and deepest desires and when we do this, we feel joy, happiness, and vitality in every moment of our existence. Situations and circumstances make life a bed of roses. Whenever we encounter a problem, we feel confident that the power within us can handle it easily. Life starts working the way we always wanted it to.

We seem to be doing the right things at the right time. The gap between our desires and their manifestation gets smaller and this happens when we have faith in the universe and do our part. Let us say you are stuck with a flat tyre and there is no one around to help you. You panic. But a car suddenly drives by, and a kind stranger helps you out.

What were the odds of that happening? This is why I believe that everything happens for a reason. Every calamity comes with a solution; you only need to believe and look for answers. None of it is a coincidence. All are just the consequences of our thoughts and actions.

Lastly, I would like to share a belief that is very close to my heart. As I mentioned earlier, believe it or not, there is something with infinite power that controls everything around us— 'The Intelligence'. It created this body and also runs it. This supreme intelligence is the generous soul which takes ten steps towards you for every single step that you take towards it.

Never ever think that the Universe is against you; it is working and supporting you all the time. Respect everyone equally. Anybody can respect a prince, but it takes a gentleman to respect a pauper. You will never speak to anyone more than you speak to yourself in your head.

So, be kind to yourself. Everything happens for a reason.

Medicine is Not Always Found in Bottles, Tablets or Vaccines

- Detoxification is Medicine.
- Quitting Junk Food is Medicine.
- Exercise is Medicine.
- Fasting is Medicine.
- Nature is Medicine
- Laughter is Medicine.
- Vegetables are Medicine.
- Sleep is Medicine.
- Sunlight is Medicine.
- Gratitude and Love are Medicine.

- Friends are Medicine.
- Meditation is Medicine.

> *Knowing is not enough; we must apply.*
> *Willing is not enough; we must do.*
> *- Johann Wolfgang von Goethe*

30

RECIPES

CONTENTS

VEGETARIAN

Chutneys | Sauces | Dips   180

18. Methi seeds chutney
19. Ridge gourd chutney
20. Red bell pepper chutney
21. Dry coconut chutney
22. Dry garlic chutney
23. Sesame pudi (Powder)
24. Walnut chutney
25. Cream avocado dip
26. Greek yogurt onion dip

Soups   187

27. Spicy pumpkin soup
28. Bottle gourd soup
29. Cream mushroom soup
30. Broccoli spinach soup
31. Broccoli cheddar soup
32. Cauliflower soup
33. Tomato soup
34. Lentil soup
35. Palak/spinach soup
36. Instant seeds porridge soup

Breakfast   195

37. Mixed dal dosa
38. Moong dosa (Pesarattu)
39. Almond cheese dosa
40. Flaxseed dosa
41. Instant dosa
42. Moong dal dosa

43. Coconut uttapam
44. Almond coconut uttapam
45. Seeds cheela
46. Seed paddu
47. Eggless cheese omelette
48. Dhokla
49. Scrambled paneer
50. Coriander vadi

Lunch| Dinner   203

51. Palak paratha
52. Paneer paratha
53. Amaranth leaves paratha
54. Cauliflower paratha
55. Coconut roti
56. Flaxseed & Groundnut roti
57. Coconut cream roti
58. Seeds roti
59. Bottle gourd talipattu
60. Nuts & seeds chapati
61. Garlic naan
62. Bhakri
63. Coconut & cauliflower rice
64. Cauliflower methi rice
65. Cauliflower palak rice
66. Cauliflower lemon rice
67. Cauliflower bisibele bath
68. Cauliflower curd rice
69. Cauliflower fried rice
70. Cauliflower poha
71. Pumpkin pulao
72. Vegetable khichdi

73. Baked veg au gratin
74. Kadhi

Bakery 225

75. Peanut butter balls
76. Laddu
77. Jamun
78. Pumpkin cheese balls
79. Flax seed bread
80. Multi seeds bread
81. Low carb bread/bun
82. 2-minute instant bread
83. Keto egg bread
84. Low carb granola bars
85. Peanut Butter Cookies
86. Lemon coconut cake
87. Brownie bites

Snacks 235

88. Ladies finger fry
89. Avocado chips
90. Low carb veg samosa
91. Almond bread cheese sandwich
92. Cabbage rolls
93. Kulfi
94. Strawberry ice-cream
95. Non-veg cutlet
96. Veg cutlet
97. Besan sev
98. Seeds mixture
99. Chakli

BREAKFAST OPTIONS

- Boiled egg with avocado smoothie
- Dhokla with pudina chutney
- Coriander vadi with mint chutney
- Besan cheela with coriander and mint chutney
- Avocado salad and Bullet coffee
- Coconut flour dosa and coconut chutney
- Almond paratha
- Mixed dal dosa with tomato chutney
- Scrambled paneer and green tea
- Cauliflower upma and coconut milk smoothie
- Sprouts with dressing/ Sprouts dosa
- Roti/ chapathi/ paratha/ idli
- Lentil rice/ Tofu rice/ Paneer rice/ Mushroom rice/ Egg rice made with diced vegetables (Cabbage | Cauliflower| Broccoli | Zucchini | Pumpkin | Ash gourd | Coconut)

LUNCH/DINNER OPTIONS (Veg/Non-veg)

- Low carb vegetable rice pulao, salad, stir fried leafy vegetables and curd
- Paneer tikka, salad, stir fried brinjal subzi and curd
- Coconut roti, palak paneer, salad, stir fried vegetables and curd
- Palak and cauliflower rice, and curd
- Cauliflower pulao, avocado salad and curd
- Cauliflower curd rice and stir-fried vegetable
- Low carb roti, chicken gravy, salad and curd
- Cauliflower rice, vegetable kurma, salad and curd
- Cabbage rice, bottle gourd dal, Sprout salad and curd
Your lunch/ dinner plate should include
- A bowl of stir-fried vegetables (stir fried with fats like cold pressed oil/ butter/ ghee)
- Protein sources like legumes/ pulses/ sprouts/ dal/ tofu/ mushroom/ paneer/ egg/ fish/ chicken/ meat preparations

- Low carb roti/ chapathi/ paratha/ dosa/ idli/ veg
- Rice made with diced cauliflower/ cabbage/ broccoli/ zucchini/ pumpkin
- A bowl of curd

SNACK OPTIONS

- Bullet coffee and nuts
- Nuts and seeds mixture
- Boiled eggs with yellow
- Jamun Fruit
- Ice Apple
- Paneer fry
- Berries
- Seed Cocktail
- Herbal Tea | Green Tea | Green Coffee
- Coffee| Tea without Sugar
- Full Fat Milk

Sugar Supplements: Stevia | Erythritol

BEVERAGES

Bulletproof coffee

Ingredients:

1 tsp instant coffee powder | 1 tsp coconut oil | pinch of cinnamon powder | 1 tsp unsalted butter

Preparation method:

1. Blend unsalted butter, coconut oil and cinnamon powder nicely
2. Add hot brewed coffee to the mixture and serve

Other options:

Fats: Virgin coconut oil, coconut butter, cocoa butter, nut butter
Flavouring: Cocoa and cocoa powder, cayenne, vanilla extract, almond extract, pepper mint extract
Add stevia or erythritol as sweetener

Serving size (ml/cup)	Energy (Kcal)	Total Carbohydrate (gm)	Fibre (gm)	Fat (gm)	Protein (gm)
100ml	46.724	4.64	0	4.64	0

Coconut milk coffee

Ingredients:

1/2 tsp instant coffee powder | 1/2 tsp stevia | 1/2 cup water 1/2 cup grated coconut

Preparation method:

1. Grind the coconut in a mixer grinder with 2 tbsp of hot water.
2. Squeeze out the coconut milk with the help of strainer and pour it in a cup and keep aside.
3. Add stevia and hot brewed coffee to the coconut milk and serve hot

Other options:

Sweetener: Erythritol
Flavour: Vanilla, peppermint, hazelnut, mint extract, cocoa powder, cinnamon, cardamom, nutmeg & dried lavender
Nut Milk: Almond, peanut, hazelnut & walnut
Seeds Milk: Sesame, flaxseed, hempseed & sunflower seed
Instead of milk use heavy whipping cream

Serving size (ml/cup)	Energy (Kcal)	Total Carbohydrate (gm)	Fibre (gm)	Fat (gm)	Protein (gm)
100 ml	286.5	12	7.2	27	2.7

Amla juice

Ingredients:

1-2 gooseberry | 1/4 tsp black salt | 200 ml of water | pinch of black pepper

Preparation method:

1. Blend chopped amla with water. Filter and discard the pulp
2. Add pepper powder and stir well.
The drink is ready to serve.

Other options:

Instead of Amla juice, you can also use lemon, aloe vera, neem, wheatgrass, ash gourd or bitter gourd.
Sweetener: Stevia or erythritol

Serving size (ml/cup)	Energy (Kcal)	Total Carbohydrate (gm)	Fibre (gm)	Fat (gm)	Protein (gm)
150ml	3.3	0.8	0.3	0.1	0.1

Tomato juice

Ingredients:

4 tomatoes | 1/4 tsp black pepper powder | celery | salt to taste

Preparation method:

1. Place an empty container beneath the nozzle of juice extractor and process the tomatoes and celery.
2. When the juicing process is complete, add salt and black pepper powder to the extracted juice and mix well.
3. Add ice cubes in serving glasses and pour juice over it.
The tomato juice is ready to serve.

Other options:

Flavour: Ginger, garlic, cinnamon, jeera, fennel, basil, cilantro
Sweetener: Stevia or erythritol
Salt: Black or Pink salt

Instead of Tomato, you can use ash gourd, bitter gourd, bottle gourd, cucumber, spinach, broccoli, parsley, kale, celery

Serving size (ml/cup)	Energy (Kcal)	Total Carbohydrate (gm)	Fibre (gm)	Fat (gm)	Protein (gm)
150ml	48	7.93	2.6	0.4	1.74

Cucumber buttermilk

Ingredients:

1/2 cup curd | 1/2 cup cucumber | 1 tsp ginger | 1/4 tsp green chilli | 2 tbsp coriander leaves | 1 tbsp curry leaves | 1 pinch of cumin powder | 1 3/4 cup water | 1/2 tsp salt

Preparation method:

1. Blend cucumber, green chilli, ginger, curry leaves and coriander leaves.

2. Add curd, salt, water, and cumin powder and blend for a while. Garnish with coriander leaves and serve chilled.

Other options

Flavour: Jeera, mint, methi, black pepper, cinnamon, asafoetida (hing), ajwain
Instead of curd, use vegan curd (almond, coconut, soya)
You can add chia seeds or flaxseeds

Serving size (ml/cup)	Energy (Kcal)	Total Carbohydrate (gm)	Fibre (gm)	Fat (gm)	Protein (gm)
150ml	167.72	8.3	2.296	4.348	5.03

Coconut shake

Ingredients:

1/2 cup unsweetened dry coconut flakes | 1/2 cup milk or coconut milk | 3/4 cup curd |1 tsp stevia | vanilla essence

Preparation method:

1. Roast the dry coconut flakes in a pan over medium heat until it turns light brown.
2. Remove the pan from the heat and transfer the roasted coconut flakes onto a plate to cool down.
3. Once cool, blend the roasted coconut flakes and add milk, vanilla essence, curd and stevia.
4. Blend until the mixture becomes smooth.
5. Transfer to a serving glass and garnish with roasted coconut flakes.
Thick coconut shake with coconut flakes is ready to serve.

Other options:

Essence: Vanilla, Peppermint, Lemon, Rose, Orange etc.
Nut Milk: Almond, Walnut
Instead of Curd, you can use yogurt or heavy whipping cream
Sweetener: Stevia or erythritol

Serving size (ml/cup)	Energy (Kcal)	Total Carbohydrate (gm)	Fibre (gm)	Fat (gm)	Protein (gm)
200ml	236.13	8.68	4.7	21.42	4.59

Green Smoothie

Ingredients:

2 tbsp spinach leaves | 1/2 avocado | 1 celery stick | 1 cup plant-based milk | 1 tbsp peanut Butter | 2 tbsp lemon juice

Preparation method:

1. Add all the ingredients to a high-speed blender.
2. Pulse to combine, stopping to scrape down the sides if necessary.
3. Blend on high speed until blended into thick and creamy consistency.
Serve immediately garnished with fresh mint.

Other options:

Sweetener: Stevia or erythritol
Other greens: Kale leaves, mint, wheat grass, lettuce, fennel stalk, celery, cilantro, parsley.
Nut Milk: Almond, peanut, hazelnut or walnut
Seeds Milk: Sesame, flaxseed, hempseed or sunflower
Fruits: Strawberry, raspberry or blueberry.
Instead of milk use Coconut cream or heavy whipped cream

Serving size (ml/cup)	Energy (Kcal)	Total Carbohydrate (gm)	Fibre (gm)	Fat (gm)	Protein (gm)
100ml	298.88	25.09	9.95	24.619	7.78

Broccoli smoothie

Ingredients:

1 cup broccoli | 1/4 cucumber | 3-4 mint leaves | 1 tsp lemon juice | 1 cup water | Pinch of salt

Preparation method:

1. Blend broccoli, cucumber, water, mint leaves and lime juice together in a blender until smooth.
Pour the smoothie in a glass and serve immediately.

Other options:

Nut Milk: Almond or coconut
Vegetables: Spinach, bottle gourd, kale, celery, wheat grass
Flavour: Cinnamon, cardamom, mint
Sweetener: Stevia or erythritol
You can add avocado or berries for flavour, and curd, yogurt or heavy whipped cream for better consistency.

Serving size (ml/cup)	Energy (Kcal)	Total Carbohydrate (gm)	Fibre (gm)	Fat (gm)	Protein (gm)
200ml	24.3	5.03	1.8	0.21	1.77

Nuts and Seeds Smoothie

Ingredients:

1 tsp flax seeds | 1 tsp pumpkin seeds | 1 tsp sunflower seeds | 1 tsp melon seeds | 1 tsp ash gourd seeds | 1 tsp cucumber seeds | 5 almonds | 2 tsp unsweetened peanut butter/ almond butter | coconut milk/ almond milk | stevia drops | pinch of cinnamon powder

Preparation method:

1. Add all seeds in a bowl (flax seeds, pumpkin seeds, sunflower seeds, melon seeds, ash gourd seeds, cucumber seeds and almonds). Soak the seeds overnight.

2. In the morning, drain off all the water and rinse, then add the seeds to the blender.
3. Add coconut milk or almond milk, peanut butter and stevia to the blender.
4. Blend it to a smooth consistency by adding water if required.
 Serve in a glass and add cinnamon powder and stir well.

Other options:

Nut Milk: Almond, peanut, hazelnut, walnut, coconut
Seeds milk: Sesame, flaxseeds, hempseed, Sunflower
Nut Butter: Almond, hazelnut, Macadamia, pecan, walnut
Seeds butter: Pumpkin, sesame, soya, sunflower
Flavour: Cocoa powder, dark chocolate, vanilla, mint or mocha
Dressing: Mixed seeds, chia seeds, cinnamon, cardamom, basil

Serving size (ml/cup)	Energy (Kcal)	Total Carbohydrate (gm)	Fibre (gm)	Fat (gm)	Protein (gm)
100ml	330.9	12.11	4.065	14.655	5.711

Chia seeds and cocoa smoothie
Ingredients:
1 1/4 cup coconut milk | 1 tbsp nut butter | 1 tbsp chia seeds | 2 tbsp cocoa powder | 1 tbsp coconut oil | pinch of cinnamon | 1/2 cup water

Preparation method:
1. Add all the ingredients into a blender.
2. Blend it to a smooth consistency by adding water if required. Garnish with cocoa powder and cinnamon and serve

Other options:

Nut Milk: Almond, peanut, hazel nut, walnut
Sweetener: Stevia or erythritol
Nut Butter: Almond, hazelnut, macadamia, pecan, walnut, brazil nut

Flavour: Dark chocolate, vanilla, mint or mocha
Dressings: Mixed seeds, mixed nuts & berries
You can add yogurt or heavy whipped cream for better consistency

Serving size (ml/cup)	Energy (Kcal)	Total Carbohydrate (gm)	Fibre (gm)	Fat (gm)	Protein (gm)
100ml	354.25	11.85	6.7	32.1	7.025

Peanut butter smoothie

Ingredients:

3 tbsp cocoa powder | 2 tbsp peanut butter | 1 cup heavy cream | 1 1/2 cups unsweetened almond milk | 6 tbsp powdered erythritol or stevia | 1/8 tsp sea salt

Preparation method:

1. Combine all the ingredients in a blender and puree until smooth. Serve in a glass and add sweetener and salt as per taste

Other options:

Milk: Nuts milk or seed milk
Nut Butter: Almond, peanut, hazelnut, walnut, pecans
Sweetener: Stevia or erythritol
Seed Butter: Pumpkin, sunflower
Essence: Cocoa, vanilla, mint or mocha
Dressings: Mixed seeds, dark chocolate, mixed nuts or berries
Instead of heavy cream, you can use coconut cream or curd

Serving size (ml/cup)	Energy (Kcal)	Total Carbohydrate (gm)	Fibre (gm)	Fat (gm)	Protein (gm)
200ml	1105	24.9	5.8	107.4	18.5

SALADS

Stir fried vegetable salad

Ingredients:

1/2 cup paneer cubes | 1/4 cup spring onions | 1 cup cauliflower | 1/2 cup capsicum | 1 cup tomatoes | 3/4 cup fenugreek leaves | pinch of black pepper powder | salt to taste | 1 tsp garam masala | 1 tsp ginger | 2 tsp ghee/ butter | pinch of mustard seeds | pinch of cumin seeds| curry leaves | pinch of hing (asafoetida)

Preparation method:

1. Heat ghee or butter in a pan, fry the paneer cubes and set aside
2. Add curry leaves, mustard seeds, cumin seeds and sauté.
3. Add ginger, spring onion, cauliflowers, turmeric and salt
4. Mix the ingredients, cover and cook until the cauliflowers are half cooked.
5. Add capsicum and tomatoes, and fry until all the vegetables are evenly cooked.
6. Sprinkle fenugreek leaves, garam masala, black pepper powder and stir properly.
Serve hot.

Other options:

Vegetables: Mushroom, baby corn, beans, broccoli, zucchini, eggplant, spinach, kale, cabbage
Flavours: Basil, oregano, cilantro
Spices: Cumin, coriander, fresh lemon grass, garlic
Sauces: Low sodium soya sauce, chilli sauce, mustard sauce
Dressing: Cream, whipping cream, virgin coconut oil, virgin olive oil, coconut flakes, Sesame seeds

Serving size (gm/cup)	Energy (Kcal)	Total Carbohydrate (gm)	Fibre (gm)	Fat (gm)	Protein (gm)
1 cup (100gm)	85.8	6.41	2.2	4.99	5.12

Stir fried vegetables with chicken

Ingredients:

1 cup chicken| 1/3 cup yellow pepper | 1/3 cup red pepper | 1/3 cup capsicum | 1 cup mushrooms | 1 cup broccoli | 1 cup baby corn | 1 cup boiled beans | 1 cup onion or spring onions |1 cup cabbage | 4 cloves garlic | 2 chopped green chillies | 2 tbsp coconut oil/ghee/ butter | pinch of salt / 2 pinches of black pepper powder

Preparation method:

1. Heat coconut oil in a pan; add chopped garlic and green chillies.
2. After a minute, add all the vegetables. Stir fry till evenly cooked.
3. Add the chicken cubes. Sprinkle salt and pepper and add soya sauce.
4. Add little water. Bring to boil and wait until properly cooked. Serve hot.

Other options:

Flavours: Basil, oregano, cilantro
Spices: Cumin, coriander, fresh lemon grass, garlic
Sauces: Low sodium soya sauce, chilli sauce, mustard sauce
Dressing: Cream, unsweetened mayonnaise, whipping cream, virgin coconut oil, virgin olive oil, coconut flakes, sesame seeds, cheese, cherry tomato, olives, peanuts
Instead of Chicken, you can use paneer, tofu, mushroom, baby corn, broccoli, zucchini.

Serving size (gm/cup)	Energy (Kcal)	Total Carbohydrate (gm)	Fibre (gm)	Fat (gm)	Protein (gm)
1 cup (100gm)	123.2	10.23	4.22	8.862	3.978

Egg salad with dressing

Ingredients:

2 boiled eggs | 1/2 avocado | 1 tbsp yogurt or curd | 1 tbsp
unsweetened mayonnaise | 1/4 tsp Dijon mustard
sauce(optional) | 1/4 tsp red chilli flakes| 2 tbsp tomatoes |
2 tbsp cucumber | 1 tsp lemon juice | pinch of salt | pinch of
chaat masala

Preparation method:

1. Cut the eggs, cucumber, avocado and tomatoes into cubes.
2. Transfer to a bowl and add chopped garlic, onion, salt, black
pepper powder, chaat masala, Dijon mustard sauce, mayonnaise
and curd.
3. Add lemon juice and mix well.
Egg salad is ready to serve

Other options:

Flavours: Parsley, ginger garlic powder, oregano, onion powder
Spices: Cumin, coriander, fresh lemon grass, garlic
Sauces: Low sodium soya sauce, chilli sauce
Dressing: Cream, heavy whipping cream, sesame seeds, cheese,
cherry tomato, olives, peanuts
Instead of Egg, you can use paneer or tofu

Serving Size (gm/cup)	Energy (Kcal)	Total Carbohydrate (gm)	Fibre (gm)	Fat (gm)	Protein (gm)
1 cup (100gm)	94.6	7.41	4	7.41	1.59

Chickpea salad

Ingredients:

100gm chickpea | 2 tbsp onion | 2 tbsp spring onions | 2 tbsp unsweetened mayonnaise | 1/4 tsp black pepper powder | 1/4 tsp red chilli powder | 1/4 tsp turmeric powder

Preparation method:

1. Soak chickpeas overnight in water and then pressure cook. Let it cool.
2. Drain and rinse the chickpeas. Transfer to a bowl.
3. Add chopped onion and spring onion.
4. Add mayonnaise, salt, pepper, red chilli powder and turmeric, and stir well.
Serve with sandwich or wrap or as a salad.

Other options:

Flavours: Parsley, ginger garlic powder, chaat masala, oregano, onion powder
Spices: Cumin, coriander
Dressing: Sesame seeds, cherry tomato
Instead of Mayonnaise, you can use heavy whipped cream, yogurt or curd

Serving size (gm/cup)	Energy (Kcal)	Total Carbohydrate (gm)	Fibre (gm)	Fat (gm)	Protein (gm)
1 cup (100gm)	375	32.3	8.9	23.8	12.8

Sautéed mushroom

Ingredients:

500g mushrooms | 3 tbsp butter/ghee |1 tsp garlic | 1/2 tsp black pepper powder| 3 tbsp fresh parsley | salt for taste

Preparation method:

1. Clean the mushrooms, slice them and set them aside.
2. Heat butter over low flame in a frying pan. Add the finely chopped garlic and sauté until fragrant for a few seconds. Add the sliced mushrooms.
3. Add freshly crushed black pepper and salt as required. Mix very well.
4. Sauté the mushroom stirring often. Initially you will see the mushrooms releasing lot of water. Gradually the water will reduce.
5. Continue to sauté until all water dries up and the mushrooms look glossy. When the water dries up, reduce heat to a low.
6. Add 1 to 3 tablespoon finely chopped parsley to taste. Mix and sauté for a minute. Taste and adjust the seasoning as required. Garnish with parsley and serve hot.

Other options:

Vegetables: Spinach, broccoli
Flavour: Garlic, butter
Dressing: Sesame seeds, Peanuts

Serving size (gm/cup)	Energy (Kcal)	Total Carbohydrate (gm)	Fibre (gm)	Fat (gm)	Protein (gm)
1 cup (100gm)	160	6.23	1.8	13.55	4.88

Stir fried broccoli with coconut

Ingredients:

2 cups broccoli |1 small onion | 2 green chillies | 1 tbsp shredded coconut | 1 tsp mustard seeds | 1/2 tsp cumin seeds | 2 tsp curry leaves | pinch of hing (asafoetida) | salt to taste | 1 tsp cold pressed coconut oil

Preparation method:

1. Heat coconut oil in a pan, temper with mustard seeds and cumin seeds, and let it splutter for a few seconds.
2. Add the green chillies, hing and curry leaves, and sauté for

another 30 seconds.

3. Now add the chopped onion and sauté till the onions are translucent and light brown.

4. Then add broccoli and salt, and stir fry on medium-low flame until soft and tender.

Garnish with fresh shredded coconut and serve.

Other options:

Other vegetables: Mushroom, pumpkin, ash gourd, spinach, squash, methi leaves, spring onions

Garnish: Parsley or cilantro or coriander leaves

Spices: Add mixed spices for flavour

Oil: Ghee or butter

Instead of small onions use spring onions

You can add coconut milk to cook the vegetables and cream for proper consistency

Serving size (gm/cup)	Energy (Kcal)	Total Carbohydrate (gm)	Fibre (gm)	Fat (gm)	Protein (gm)
1 cup (100gm)	375	32.3	8.9	23.8	12.8

CHUTNEYS/SAUCES/ DIPS

Methi seeds chutney

Ingredients:

1 tbsp fenugreek seeds | 3 garlic cloves | 1 tsp curry leaves | 1 cup grated coconut | 2 tsp tamarind pulp | 1 tsp cumin seeds | 2 tbsp red chilli powder | 1/2 cup water | salt to taste

Preparation method:

1. Dry roast fenugreek seeds before grinding into a powder.
2. Add all the other ingredients and grind it into a smooth paste. Serve the methi chutney with idli or dosa.

Serving size (tsp/tbsp)	Energy (Kcal)	Total Carbohydrate (gm)	Fibre (gm)	Fat (gm)	Protein (gm)
1 tbsp	94	9.78	6.4	5.44	2.81

Ridge gourd chutney

Ingredients:

1 cup ridge gourd with skin | 1 tsp urad dal | 2 green chillies | ½ inch tamarind | 3 cloves garlic | 1/2 tsp coconut oil | 1/2 tsp mustard seeds | 5-6 curry leaves | 1 pinch of hing (asafoetida) | salt for taste

Preparation method:

1. Add oil in a pan and place over medium flame. Once the oil is hot, add urad dal and fry till it turns light brown.
2. Then add green chillies, garlic, tamarind, sauté for another 1 minute
3. Cool it and put it in a blender.
3. Now fry the chopped ridge gourd in ½ teaspoon of oil until it turns light brown. Keep it aside until it cools down.

4. Then grind everything together along with salt into a fine paste. Add the tempering to the chutney and serve with idli or dosa.

Other options

Vegetables: Mint leaves, brahmi leaves, methi leaves, curry leaves, Coriander leaves.

Serving size (tsp/tbsp)	Energy (Kcal)	Total Carbohydrate (gm)	Fibre (gm)	Fat (gm)	Protein (gm)
1 tbsp	105.46	12.299	3.88	5.102	4.034

Red bell pepper chutney

Ingredients:

1 large red bell pepper | 1/2 medium-sized onion | 2 cloves garlic | 5 dried red chillies | 1/2 inch of tamarind | 1/4 cup peanuts | 1/2 tsp coconut oil | 1/2 tsp mustard seeds | 5-6 curry leaves | pinch of Hing (asafoetida) | salt to taste

Preparation method:

1. Heat coconut oil in a pan.
2. Add garlic, dried red chillies, curry leaves and onions, and sauté for about 1-2 minutes until onions become soft.
3. Add red bell pepper and sauté till soft. Remove from heat and allow to cool.
4. Roast peanuts until golden brown. Let them cool down.
5. In a blender, add the roasted bell pepper-onion mixture, roasted peanuts, tamarind and salt. Grind them together to a coarse or smooth paste by adding little water.
Red bell pepper chutney is ready to serve.

Other options

Vegetables: *Tomato, brinjal, green chilli, ladies finger*

Serving size (tsp/tbsp)	Energy (Kcal)	Total Carbohydrate (gm)	Fibre (gm)	Fat (gm)	Protein (gm)
1 tbsp	117.4	8.05	13.32	9.482	1.69

Dry coconut chutney powder

Ingredients:

1/2 cup grated dry coconut | 3 garlic cloves | 3-4 dry chillies | 2 tbsp chana dal | 1 tsp urad dal | 1/2 tsp coconut oil | salt to taste.

Preparation method:

1. Roast the dry red chillies, urad dal, and chana dal until light brown in coconut oil.
Transfer to a plate and allow it to cool.
2. Roast the grated coconut and garlic for a minute over low flame in the same pan. Turn off the flame, transfer to a plate, and allow them to cool.
3. Grind all the roasted ingredients into a powder along with salt. Do not make the powder very smooth. It should have a coarse texture.
Dry coconut chutney powder can be served with any meal.

Other options

Instead of dry coconut, you can use peanuts or bengal gram.

Serving size (tsp/tbsp)	Energy (Kcal)	Total Carbohydrate (gm)	Fibre (gm)	Fat (gm)	Protein (gm)
1 tbsp	154.14	15.59	2.12	4.1	9.66

Dry garlic chutney

Ingredients:

8 garlic cloves |1/2 cup grated dry coconut | 1 tbsp sesame seeds | 1 tbsp peanuts | 2 tsp red chilli powder | 1 tsp coriander powder | 1/2 tsp tamarind paste | 1 tsp coconut oil | salt for taste

Preparation method:

1. Heat 1 tsp oil in pan and roast garlic cloves over low flame for 1 minute. Turn off flame and transfer it to a plate.
2. Dry roast grated coconut in same pan until light brown.
3. Dry roast sesame seeds over low flame until seeds start to pop and transfer to a plate.
4. Cool the roasted garlic, roasted coconut and sesame seeds for 5 minutes. Add roasted peanuts, tamarind paste, red chilli powder, coriander powder and salt.
5. Grind the ingredients to a medium coarse powder.
Serve the chutney or transfer to an air tight container.

Serving size (tsp/tbsp)	Energy (Kcal)	Total Carbohydrate (gm)	Fibre (gm)	Fat (gm)	Protein (gm)
1 tbsp	175.9	12.9	2	3.2	13.45

Sesame pudi (Powder)

Ingredients:

100gm sesame seeds | 1/2 tbsp ghee | 15 dry red chilli | 1/4 cup curry leaves | 1 tsp asafoetida | 100gm desiccated coconut | 50gm roasted peanut | salt for taste

Preparation method:

1. Roast all the ingredients in ghee until they turn golden brown.
2. Grind them into a coarse powder.
Serve the pudi with dosa or idli

Other options

Instead of Sesame seeds, you can use flax seeds, peanuts or bengal gram.

Serving size (tsp/tbsp)	Energy (Kcal)	Total Carbohydrate (gm)	Fibre (gm)	Fat (gm)	Protein (gm)
1 tbsp	180.9	6.524	1.8	15.04	3.314

Walnut Chutney

Ingredients:

2 tbsp walnuts | 1/2 cup grated fresh coconut | 2 green chillies | 1 inch ginger | 1 tsp tamarind pulp | 1 tsp curry leaves | 1 tbsp coriander leaves | 1 tsp coconut oil | 1 tsp mustard oil |1/2 tsp urad dal | pinch of hing (asafoetida) | salt for taste

Preparation method:

1. In a mixer jar, add the freshly grated coconut, raw walnuts, green chillies, ginger, coriander leaves, curry leaves, tamarind and salt. Grind to a fine paste using some water.
2. Heat a little oil in a pan, add mustard seeds, split urad dal, hing and curry leaves.
3. Sauté for a few seconds until the urad dal turns light brown.
4. Pour this tempering over the chutney paste and mix well.
Serve the walnut chutney with idli and dosa.

Serving size (tsp/tbsp)	Energy (Kcal)	Total Carbohydrate (gm)	Fibre (gm)	Fat (gm)	Protein (gm)
1 tbsp	114.7	9.014	1.332	8.66	2.5

Creamy avocado dip

Ingredients:

2 ripe avocados |1/2 cup plain greek yogurt | 2 chopped cloves of garlic | juice of 1 lime | salt to taste | black pepper powder | vegetable sticks for serving

Preparation method:

1. In a medium bowl, mash avocados with a fork.
2. Stir in the yogurt, garlic, lime juice and season generously with salt and pepper.
Serve with vegetables sticks.

Other options

Flavours: Cilantro or parsley
Yogurt: Cream or cheese

Serving size (tsp/tbsp)	Energy (Kcal)	Total Carbohydrate (gm)	Fibre (gm)	Fat (gm)	Protein (gm)
1 tbsp	33.3	2.34	1.06	2.23	1.27

Greek yogurt onion dip

Ingredients:

2 cups greek yogurt | 2 thinly sliced onions | 2 tbsp butter | freshly ground pepper | 1 tsp apple cider vinegar | nut crackers for serving| salt to taste

Preparation method:

1. Heat butter in a skillet over medium heat.
2. Add the onions. Turn down the heat to medium-low and cook for about 20 minutes, stirring occasionally, until the onions are soft and caramelized.
3. If the onions are browning too quickly, turn down the heat and add a splash of water.
4. When the onions are caramelized, add vinegar and cook for

about 1 minute until the vinegar reduces slightly. Remove from heat.

5. In a medium serving bowl, combine the caramelized onions and Greek yogurt.

6. Season to taste with salt and pepper

Serve cold with carrot sticks and nut crackers.

Other options

Flavour: Cilantro, parsley or lemon grass

Garnish for dips: Spring onions, caramelized onions, bell peppers, red onions or chopped garlic.

Spices: Paprika, chilli powder, cayenne pepper

Serving size (tsp/tbsp)	Energy (Kcal)	Total Carbohydrate (gm)	Fibre (gm)	Fat (gm)	Protein (gm)
1 tbsp	71.3	4.9	0.66	5.18	0.6

SOUPS

Spicy pumpkin soup

1 cup pumpkin |1 tbsp butter| 90 ml fresh cream | 1 onion | 1/2 tbsp red chilli powder | 1/2 tsp coriander leaves | 1 tsp black pepper | 1/2 tsp cumin powder | 1 garlic clove | salt to taste

Preparation method:

1. Cook onion in butter in a pan over medium heat for 3-4 minutes or until soft.
2. Add garlic, cumin powder, and red chilli powder and cook for 1 minute longer.
3. Add pumpkin to the pan, bring to boil, then reduce heat and simmer for 15-20 minutes or until pumpkin is tender. Remove pan from the heat and set aside to cool.
4. Blend all the ingredients into a soup like consistency.
5. Pour the soup to a clean saucepan, add cream, salt as per taste, black pepper and heat over a medium flame, without boiling. Garnish with coriander leaves and serve hot.

Serving size (ml/cup)	Energy (Kcal)	Total Carbohydrate (gm)	Fibre (gm)	Fat (gm)	Protein (gm)
150 ml	314.2	9.69	1.2	30.036	2.12

Bottle gourd soup

Ingredients:

1 medium bottle gourd/lauki | 1 tsp coconut oil | 3 chopped medium garlic cloves | 1 green chilli | 1 medium-sized onion | 1 ½ cups water | salt and black pepper to taste | coriander leaves

Preparation method:

1. Add coconut oil in a pan and place it on medium heat.
2. Once the oil is hot, add chopped garlic, onions and green chilli, and sauté until onions soften.
3. Add diced bottle-gourd, water or vegetable stock, and salt.
4. Cover with a lid and cook for 5 minutes.
5. Once cooked, let it cool down for 5-10 minutes, and puree in a blender.
6. Add salt and crushed black pepper for seasoning.
7. If soup is too thick, add some water or vegetable stock and boil for 2 minutes.
Garnish with coriander leaves and serve the bottle gourd soup.

Other options

Flavour: Parsley, celery, cilantro
Vegetables: Ridge gourd, squash, tomato, ash gourd, pumpkin

Serving size (ml/cup)	Energy (Kcal)	Total Carbohydrate (gm)	Fibre (gm)	Fat (gm)	Protein (gm)
150 ml	286	10.99	1	26.16	1.89

Cream of mushroom soup

Ingredients:

3 cups diced mushroom |1 tbsp coconut oil | 2 tbsp onion | 3 cloves garlic | 1/2 cup celery | 2 cups water or vegetable stock | 1/2 cup coconut cream | salt & black pepper to taste | 2 tbsp coriander leaves | 2 tbsp cream

Preparation method:

1. To a pan, add coconut oil, onion, garlic, and sauté till onions soften.
2. Then add diced mushrooms and celery, and sauté till all the liquid that is released from the mushroom has evaporated. This will take about 6-8 minutes.
3. Add water or vegetable stock, salt and black pepper powder. Mix

well.
4. Add all the ingredients to a pressure cooker and cook on high pressure for 5 minutes.
5. Allow to cool down and then puree in a blender.
6. Add coconut cream or heavy cream to the puree and stir well. If the consistency is too thick, add water or coconut milk and simmer for 2 minutes.
Garnish with coriander leaves and serve hot.

Flavour: Parsley or Celery

Serving size (ml/cup)	Energy (Kcal)	Total Carbohydrate (gm)	Fibre (gm)	Fat (gm)	Protein (gm)
150 ml	306	6.83	0.915	29.9	2.46

Broccoli spinach soup

Ingredients:

1 cup broccoli | 1 cup spinach | 1 tbsp chopped garlic | 1/2 cup onion | 1 tbsp butter | 1/2 cup almond milk or coconut milk | 1 cup water or vegetable stock | 1/4 cup mozzarella cheese | 1/4 tsp black pepper powder | salt to taste

Preparation method:

1. Add butter in a pan and place on medium heat.
2. Once the butter melts, add chopped garlic and sauté for 30 seconds.
3. Add onions and sauté till they turn translucent.
4. Then add broccoli and water, stir and cook in a pressure cooker.
5. Let it cool down for 5 minutes.
6. Add spinach, cheese, milk, salt, and pepper to taste. Stir well.
7. Puree in a blender and transfer the soup to a vessel and boil for 2 minutes, until it gets a thick consistency.
Garnish and serve the broccoli spinach soup hot.

Other options

Flavour: Tulsi, garlic, parsley, spring onions, fresh herbs

Serving size (ml/cup)	Energy (Kcal)	Total Carbohydrate (gm)	Fibre (gm)	Fat (gm)	Protein (gm)
150 ml	288	10.74	2.5	18.16	5.77

Broccoli cheddar soup

Ingredients:

3 cups fresh broccoli | 2 tbsp butter |1 cup onion | 3 cloves garlic | 1/2 cup shredded carrots | 2 cups water | 2 tbsp besan (chickpea) flour | 2 cups cheddar cheese | 1 cup milk or cream |salt and pepper to taste

Preparation method:

1. Melt butter in a pan over medium flame. Add minced garlic, diced onions, and sauté till the onions turn translucent.
2. Add the flour and sauté for a minute, stirring constantly, until it is cooked.
3. Then add the shredded carrot, chopped broccoli, salt, crushed black pepper, and water, and give it a stir.
4. Cook everything in a pressure cooker.
5. Let it cool down for 5 minutes.
6. Puree in the blender till it becomes a fine paste.
7. Add milk and cheddar cheese to the puree and stir for 2-3 minutes until the cheese melts.
8. Add salt and pepper and let the soup simmer for 2 minutes. Garnish and serve broccoli cheddar soup hot.

Serving size (ml/cup)	Energy (Kcal)	Total Carbohydrate (gm)	Fibre (gm)	Fat (gm)	Protein (gm)
150 ml	302.82	13.26	2.5	18.3	6.03

Cauliflower soup

3 cups cauliflower|1 cup onion | 4 garlic cloves | 1 tbsp butter | 1 bay leaf | 2 cups water |1/2 cup coconut cream (or coconut milk) | ¼ tsp black pepper | 2-3 tsp cheddar cheese |1/4 tsp oregano | salt to taste

Preparation method:

1. Add butter in a pan and place it on medium flame. Add bay leaf, chopped garlic and onion, and sauté until they soften.
2. Add cauliflower, water or vegetable stock, black pepper powder, and salt.
3. Cook the above ingredients in a pressure cooker.
4. Remove the bay leaf and puree the mixture in the blender to make a fine paste.
5. Allow it to cool.
6. Add heavy cream and cheese, and stir well.
7. If the soup is too thick, you can add water or milk and boil it for 2 minutes.
Garnish with green onions, oregano, and more cheese, and serve hot.

Serving size (ml/cup)	Energy (Kcal)	Total Carbohydrate (gm)	Fibre (gm)	Fat (gm)	Protein (gm)
150 ml	301	8.96	1.5	20.8	4.37

Tomato soup

3 cups tomatoes | 1 cup onion | 1/2 red bell pepper | 3 cloves garlic | 1 tbsp butter or coconut oil | 2 cups water or vegetable stock | 1 bay leaf | 2 tsp basil | salt & black pepper powder for taste | 1/4 cup heavy cream/milk

Preparation method:

1. Heat butter or oil over a low flame in a pan. Add bay leaf, chopped garlic and onions, and sauté until they soften.
2. Add red bell pepper, diced tomatoes, water or vegetable stock, black pepper powder, and salt.
3. Cook everything in a pressure cooker.
4. Let it cool down.
5. Remove the bay leaf and puree everything in a blender to make a fine paste.
6. Add dried basil and heavy cream and stir well.
7. If the soup is too thick, add water or milk and boil for 2 minutes.

Drizzle a bit of heavy cream and serve the tomato soup hot.

Serving size (ml/cup)	Energy (Kcal)	Total Carbohydrate (gm)	Fibre (gm)	Fat (gm)	Protein (gm)
150 ml	110.7	8.4	1.81	8.43	1.61

Lentil soup

Ingredients:

3 cups whole green lentil | 1 tbsp coconut oil | 1 cup chopped onion | 1 cup chopped tomatoes | 3 cloves garlic | 1/2 cup celery | 1/2 cup red bell pepper | 1/2 tsp crushed black pepper | 3 cups water | 1/2 cup coconut milk | 2-3 cups cut baby spinach | 2 tbsp lemon juice | 2 tsp garam masala powder | 1/2 tsp turmeric powder | 1/2 tsp red chilli powder |1 tsp cumin powder | salt to taste

Preparation method:

1. Wash and thoroughly rinse the lentil.
2. Heat oil in a pan, add chopped garlic and sauté for 30 seconds.
3. Add onions and sauté until they soften.
4. Add celery, red bell pepper, tomatoes, and green lentils into the pan.
5. Then add dry spice powders like turmeric, ground cumin, red

chilli, and garam masala into the pan. Add vegetable stock or water.
6. Add salt and black pepper and cook in a pressure cooker.
7. Allow it to cool down.
8. Add lemon juice and baby spinach. Keep stirring until the spinach wilts.
Garnish and serve the green lentil soup warm.

Other options

Herbs: Celery, parsley, cilantro
Instead of green lentils, you can use masoor dal, toor dal, Chickpeas or horsegram

Serving size (ml/cup)	Energy (Kcal)	Total Carbohydrate (gm)	Fibre (gm)	Fat (gm)	Protein (gm)
150 ml	281.5	29.133	8.351	6.495	9.26

Palak/Spinach soup

Ingredients:

1 cup palak/ spinach | 1 cinnamon sticks | 1 tomato | 1/2 tbsp butter/ghee | 1 onion | 5gm ginger | 1 tsp cumin powder |1/4 black pepper powder |1/4 tsp salt | 2 cups water

Preparation method:

1. Chop onion, tomato, spinach /palak and ginger.
2. In a pressure cooker, heat butter and add cinnamon stick, chopped onions and ginger. Fry till the onions turn translucent.
3. Add chopped tomatoes and chopped spinach/palak leaves along with salt, pepper powder, cumin powder and coriander powder. Sauté for a few minutes.
4. Add a little water and pressure cook.
5. Cool this mixture and grind it.
6. Pour the blended mixture in a pan along with some water and let this simmer for a few minutes.
Garnish and serve the palak soup warm

Other options
Herbs: Celery, oregano, parsley or cilantro
Butter: Ghee, cold pressed coconut oil
Instead of water, you can use cream, whipping cream or coconut milk

Serving size (ml/cup)	Energy (Kcal)	Total Carbohydrate (gm)	Fibre (gm)	Fat (gm)	Protein (gm)
150 ml	161.8	9.98	4.09	5.3	2.81

Instant seeds porridge soup

Ingredients:
1/4 cup curd | 1 tbsp chia seeds | 2 tbsp pumpkin seeds | 2 tbsp flaxseeds | 1 tbsp chopped onions | 2 tbsp water melon seeds | 2 cup warm water | salt to taste

Preparation method:
1. To make instant mix, dry roast the flaxseeds, watermelon seeds and pumpkin seeds on low flame. Add chia seeds after turning off the flame.
2. Allow to cool and grind roasted seeds into a fine powder. Store it in an air-tight container.
3. To make the soup, add 2 cups of warm water to the porridge mix in a bowl.
4. Add chopped onion, whisked curd, and salt.

Other options
Garnish: Sunflower seeds, pumpkin seeds, sesame seeds, flaxseeds, ghee, butter
Instead of warm water, you can use cream, almond milk or coconut milk

Serving size (ml/cup)	Energy (Kcal)	Total Carbohydrate (gm)	Fibre (gm)	Fat (gm)	Protein (gm)
150 ml	268.5	21.71	7.17	9.66	8.2

BREAKFAST

Mixed dal dosa

Ingredients:

3 cups moong dal | 2 cups urad dal | 1 cup chana dal | 1 ¼ tsp jeera | 1 ¼ tsp chilli powder | 1 ¼ tsp grated ginger | pinch of turmeric powder | 2 tbsp chopped coriander leaves | 1 tbsp grated cabbage | 1 tbsp chopped capsicum | 1 tbsp coconut oil | salt for taste

Preparation method:

1. Add all the dals to a blender and blend to make mixed gram flour.
2. To 2 cups of mixed gram flour, add jeera, grated ginger, chilli powder, turmeric powder, chopped coriander, capsicum and cabbage.
3. Mix all the ingredients well with sufficient water, and leave it aside for 10 minutes.
4. Grease a dosa pan with coconut oil. Pour the batter on it and allow it to cook completely for 2 minutes on low heat.
5. Cover and cook on one side and flip.
Serve the mixed dal dosa hot, with chutney.

Serving size (pieces/no)	Energy (Kcal)	Total Carbohydrate (gm)	Fibre (gm)	Fat (gm)	Protein (gm)
2 no	185.17	26.65	9.80	7.998	9.148

Moong dosa (Pesarattu)

Ingredients:

Green gram 1 cup | 2 red chillies | 1 tsp grated ginger | 1 chopped onion | 2 tbsp chopped coriander leaves | 1 tsp coconut oil | salt to taste

Preparation method:

1. Soak green gram overnight and in the morning, grind it with chillies, ginger and salt. Add chopped onions and coriander leaves.
2. Grease the pan with coconut oil and pour the batter. Allow it to cook completely on low heat. Cover and cook on one side and flip. Serve the moong dal dosa hot with chutney.

You can use 1 tsp of gondu as thickening or binding agent

Serving size (pieces/no)	Energy (Kcal)	Total Carbohydrate (gm)	Fibre (gm)	Fat (gm)	Protein (gm)
2 no	32.5	8.64	1.874	0.208	2.74

Almond cheese dosa

Ingredients:

20 Almonds | 2 slices cheese | 1/4 cup water | 1 cup coconut milk | 1 tsp butter | 2 tsp ghee | salt for taste

Preparation method:

1. Soak the almonds for 10 minutes in hot water.
2. Grind the almonds and coconut milk into a smooth batter.
3. Dissolve cheese in a little warm water. Mix the cheese and salt into batter.
4. Heat a non-stick tawa on low heat. Ladle out the batter, spread it over tawa, cover and cook on one side and flip.
Serve the almond cheese dosa hot with chutney.

Serving size (pieces/no)	Energy (Kcal)	Total Carbohydrate (gm)	Fibre (gm)	Fat (gm)	Protein (gm)
2 no	219.49	2.95	1.6	6.9	20.84

Flaxseed dosa

2 tbsp chia seeds | 1 tbsp coconut oil | 50g almonds | 100g whole flaxseeds | salt for taste

Preparation method:

1. Soak the almonds and flaxseeds for 3 hours.
2. Grind the chia seeds into a fine powder.
3. Peel the almond skin and grind it into a paste.
4. Grind the soaked flaxseed and transfer all the ground ingredients into a bowl. Add ½ cup of water and salt to get the batter consistency. Allow it to ferment for 2 hours.
5. Grease the tawa with coconut oil and pour the batter. Allow it to cook completely for 2 minutes on low heat and flip.
Serve the flax seed dosa hot with coconut chutney.

You can use 1 tsp of gondu as thickening or binding agent

Serving size (pieces/no)	Energy (Kcal)	Total Carbohydrate (gm)	Fibre (gm)	Fat (gm)	Protein (gm)
2 no	180	8.19	6.2	15.33	5.01

Instant dosa

Ingredients:

4 tsp chia seeds | 1 ½ tsp coconut oil | 2 tbsp pumpkin seeds | 2 tbsp whole flaxseed | 2 tbsp watermelon seeds | salt for taste

Preparation method:

1. Heat a pan on low flame and dry roast the flax seeds, melon seeds, and pumpkin seeds. Turn off the heat and add chia seeds.
2. Allow the roasted seeds to cool for 2 minutes and grind into a fine powder.
3. Add salt and water to the seed mix.

4. Heat a non-stick tawa on low flame. Take batter and spread it over the tawa. Sprinkle oil on the dosa batter. Cover the tawa with a lid and cook.

5. Repeat previous step with the remaining batter.

Serve the instant dosa hot, with chutney.

Serving size (pieces/no)	Energy (Kcal)	Total Carbohydrate (gm)	Fibre (gm)	Fat (gm)	Protein (gm)
2 no	163	3.9	3	15.8	7.8

Moong dal dosa

Ingredients:

Moong dal 1 cup | 2-3 green chillies | 1 tsp garlic | 1 tsp ginger |1 tbsp ghee/butter | salt to taste

Preparation method:

1. Soak the moong dal overnight.

2. In the morning, grind the moong dal in a blender along with chillies, garlic, ginger, salt and water, till it is a smooth paste.

3. Heat a non-stick pan on medium flame. Ladle out the batter and spread it over the tawa.

4. Sprinkle some ghee and cook the dosa on both sides.

5. Cover and cook on one side and flip.

Serve the Moong dal dosa hot, with chutney.

Other options

Instead of ghee, you can use butter or cold pressed coconut oil.

For thickening/binding add gondu or xanthan gum

Serving size (pieces/no)	Energy (Kcal)	Total Carbohydrate (gm)	Fibre (gm)	Fat (gm)	Protein (gm)
2 no	156	10.126	2.454	11.5	3.75

Coconut uttapam

Ingredients:

1-2 cup grated coconut | 1 tbsp coconut oil | 1 tbsp milk cream | 1 tbsp chia seeds | 1 chopped onion | 2 chopped green chillies | 1 tbsp peanut | 1 tbsp butter | 1 tbsp curry leaves | salt to taste

Preparation method:

1. Grind coconut into a fine paste.
2. Grind chia seeds and 1 tbsp of peanuts into fine powder.
3. Add coconut paste, chia seed powder, chopped onion, chillies, curry leaves, butter, groundnut powder, salt into a bowl and mix it into a batter consistency.
4. Cover the bowl and let the batter rest for 20 minutes.
5. Heat the tawa, pour some oil and spread the batter.
6. Keep in low flame and cook uttapam on both sides.
Serve the coconut uttapam warm with chutney.

Other options

Instead of ghee, you can use butter or cold pressed coconut oil.
For thickening/binding, you can add gondu or xanthan gum

Serving size (pieces/no)	Energy (Kcal)	Total Carbohydrate (gm)	Fibre (gm)	Fat (gm)	Protein (gm)
2 no	340	14.76	8.7	31.27	4.03

Almond coconut uttapam

Ingredients:

1/2 cup shredded coconut | 1 tbsp coconut oil | 20 g almonds | 2 tsp raw chia seeds | salt for taste

Preparation method:

1. Soak the almonds for 10 minutes in hot water.
2. Grind the almond, coconut and chia seeds into a fine paste with salt.

3. Batter should be of thick consistency.
4. Heat a tawa on medium flame and spread some coconut oil.
5. Scoop a portion of the batter and spread it on the pan.
6. Cook the uttapam on both sides.
Serve the almond coconut uttapam with mint kurma

Other options

For thickening add gondu or xanthan gum
Garnish: Cilantro, spring onions
Toppings: Mozzarella cheese (shredded cheese) or cottage cheese

Serving size (pieces/no)	Energy (Kcal)	Total Carbohydrate (gm)	Fibre (gm)	Fat (gm)	Protein (gm)
2 no	165.3	7.19	5.11	14.58	3.46

Seeds cheela

Ingredients:

3 tbsp sunflower seeds | 3 tbsp sesame seeds | 1/4 tsp
turmeric | 2 tsp butter | half tomato | 3 tbsp cheese | 5
almonds | 2 tbsp chopped onions | 1/2 tsp ginger | pinch of
hing | 1/2 tsp ajwain | salt to taste

Preparation method:

1. Warm a pan over medium heat. Dry roast sunflower seeds and
sesame seeds.
2. Grind roasted seeds, almond and water into smooth batter.
3. Add finely chopped onions, tomatoes, ajwain, turmeric powder,
ginger, cheese, coriander leaves and salt to the batter and mix well.
4. Warm a non-stick tawa on low heat. Ladle out the batter, spread
it over the tawa, and spread some butter on the cheela. Cover the
tawa with a lid and cook for 3 minutes.
Serve seeds cheela warm, with chutney.

Other options
Instead of butter, you can use ghee or coconut oil

Serving size (pieces/no)	Energy (Kcal)	Total Carbohydrate (gm)	Fibre (gm)	Fat (gm)	Protein (gm)
2 no	367	12.96	3.71	34.08	6.265

Seeds paddu

Ingredients:

1/4 cup sunflower seeds | 1/2 tbsp chia seeds | 1/2 tbsp coconut oil | 2 green chilli | 1 pinch baking soda |5-6 curry leaves |2 tbsp curd | 1/2 cup chopped onions | 1/2 tbsp watermelon seeds | salt to taste

Preparation method:

1. Grind sunflower seeds, melon seeds and chia seeds into fine powder. Mix the ground powder, curd, baking soda, 1 tbsp water and salt.
2. Add the chopped green chilli, onion, curry leaves and mix well to form dosa batter consistency. Let the batter rest for 10 minutes.
3. Heat the paddu tawa, apply some oil and pour the batter. Cover and cook on both sides on low flame.
Serve seeds paddu, warm with chutney.

Other options

For improving the consistency of the batter, you can add psyllium husk, gondu or xanthan gum. To the Seeds batter you can also add methi seeds powder, paneer, egg white, tofu and cheese.

Serving size (pieces/no)	Energy (Kcal)	Total Carbohydrate (gm)	Fibre (gm)	Fat (gm)	Protein (gm)
4 no	258.3	12.29	5.81	21.81	6.83

Eggless cheese omelette

Ingredients:

1/4 tsp salt | 1/2 bell pepper |1/2 tomato | 1/4 cup beans | 1 tbsp coconut oil | 2 tbsp onion | 4 slice cheddar-cheese | 1 green chilli | 1/4 tsp black pepper powder|25 g cucumber (optional)

Preparation method:

1. Take a mixing bowl and add tomato, onion, green chilli, beans, bell pepper and grated cucumber.
2. Add salt and black pepper powder as per taste, bring the mixture to batter consistency.
3. Heat the pan and add coconut oil, spread the vegetable mixture along with cheese.
4. Cook on medium flame, flip over and cook the other side as well.
Eggless cheese omelette is ready to serve

For thickening/binding agent, you can use besan flour and gondu

Serving size (pieces/no)	Energy (Kcal)	Total Carbohydrate (gm)	Fibre (gm)	Fat (gm)	Protein (gm)
2 no	273.3	9.57	1.2	24.43	4.45

Dhokla

Ingredients:

20 almonds | 1/2 cup besan flour| 9 tbsp watermelon seeds | 1 tbsp curry leaves | 1/4 tsp lemon juice | pinch of asafoetida (hing) | 1/2 tbsp coconut oil | 1/2 tsp ghee | 1/4 tsp mustard seeds | a pinch of turmeric powder | 3 tbsp curd | pinch of baking soda | 1/4 tsp salt

Preparation method:

1. Soak the almonds in water for 10 minutes. Drain and peel off the skin.

2. In a separate bowl, soak the melon seeds in 3 tbsp of water for 10 minutes. Do not dry.

3. Grind melon seeds along with the soaking water and the almonds until the mixture reaches a semolina like consistency.

4. In a bowl, add the seeds mixture, yogurt, salt, turmeric powder, lemon juice, and baking soda. Mix well.

5. Heat an idli cooker with 1-2 glass of water over medium heat. Grease an idli plate with ghee, pour the batter, and cook for 15 minutes.

6. Once the dhokla is cooked, remove from the plate and cut into pieces.

7. Tempering - Heat coconut oil in a pan over medium flame and add mustard seeds. When the seeds start popping, add asafoetida (hing) and curry leaves.

Pour the tempering over the dhokla and serve warm with mint chutney.

Other options

Instead of coconut oil, you can use ghee or butter

Serving size (pieces/no)	Energy (Kcal)	Total Carbohydrate (gm)	Fibre (gm)	Fat (gm)	Protein (gm)
4 no	181.8	10.0	5.316	14.18	4.406

Scrambled paneer

Ingredients:

250g Paneer | 1 cup chopped tomatoes | 3 tbsp butter | 1/2 cup chopped onion | 1 slice ginger | 4 garlic cloves | 2 chopped green chillies | 1/2 tsp garam masala powder | 1/2 tsp coriander powder | 1/2 tsp red chilli powder | 3 tbsp chopped coriander leaves |1 tsp salt | 1/4 tsp turmeric powder | 1/2 tsp cumin seeds

Preparation method:

1. Crumble the Paneer (cottage cheese) and keep aside.

2. Crush the ginger and garlic to a paste and keep aside. Keep the

spice powders aside.

3. Heat butter in a pan on a medium-low flame.

4. Add cumin seeds. Once it crackles and changes colour (becomes brown) add the onions.

5. When the onions become translucent, add the ginger-garlic paste and chopped green chillies.

6. Now add the tomatoes and sauté on medium-low heat till they become soft. You can add a pinch of salt to make the tomatoes cook faster.

7. Add all the dry spice powders - turmeric, red chilli powder, coriander powder, and garam masala powder.

8. Mix the spice powders very well and sauté for 5-6 seconds.

9. Then add the crumbled Paneer. Mix thoroughly and cook for one minute. Don't cook paneer for a long time as they can become hard or rubbery.

Garnish with chopped coriander and serve hot.

Other options

Flavour: Mixed herbs, basil, mint or oregano

Instead of butter, you can use coconut oil or ghee

Serving size (gm/cup)	Energy (Kcal)	Total Carbohydrate (gm)	Fibre (gm)	Fat (gm)	Protein (gm)
1 cup (100 gm)	130.6	10.37	1.754	6.49	8.54

Coriander Vadi

Ingredients:

2 tbsp besan flour | 2 tbsp sesame seeds | 1 tsp garam masala | salt to taste | 1/2 tsp turmeric powder | 1 cup coriander leaves | 1/4 cup water | 2 tbsp coconut oil

Preparation method:

1. Chop the coriander leaves into small pieces.

2. Mix all the ingredients and spread it on a greased plate. Steam for 15 min.

3. After steaming, allow it to cool down for 5 min.
4. Cut it into desired shape and size.
5. Heat coconut oil in a pan over medium flame.
6. Add the coriander vadi pieces and shallow fry on both sides until golden and serve hot.

Serving size (pieces/no)	Energy (Kcal)	Total Carbohydrate (gm)	Fibre (gm)	Fat (gm)	Protein (gm)
4 no	184	12.44	5.6	12.88	6.06

LUNCH / DINNER

Palak paratha

Ingredients:

2 cup- low carb flour| 1 ½ cup palak/ spinach | 2-3 green chilli | 1 tsp Jeera | 1 tsp ajwain | salt for taste | 1 cup water | 1 tbsp ghee

Preparation method:

1. In a blender add palak/ spinach, green chilli, jeera and salt. Grind it into a fine smooth paste.
2. Mix all the ingredients in a bowl. Knead the flour with palak mix and make into balls.
3. Take two parchment papers, place the dough in between and roll thinly to round shape.
4. Heat a tawa on medium flame, and place the paratha on it.
5. Sprinkle some ghee and cook on both sides.
Serve the hot paratha with chutney.
In addition to low-carb flour, you may also use Coconut flour or almond flour or nuts & seeds flour

Serving size (pieces/no)	Energy (Kcal)	Total Carbohydrate (gm)	Fibre (gm)	Fat (gm)	Protein (gm)
2 no	330	21.64	11.114	16.22	25.22

Paneer paratha

Ingredients:

200g paneer | 1/2 cup onion | 2-3 green chilli | 2 tbsp coriander leaves | 1 tsp jeera | 200g low carb flour| 2 tsp coconut oil | salt for taste

Preparation method:

1. Grate or finely crumble the paneer.
2. Sauté the onions, green chilli and jeera for 2 min. Add paneer

and mix nicely.
3. Make small balls out of the paneer mix.
4. Make dough of low carb high protein flour atta or plain atta or coconut flour.
5. Let the dough rest for 30 min. Divide it into small balls.
6. Roll out a ball of the dough. Place the paneer mix in the centre. Seal the edges and roll it out once again.
7. Place the paneer paratha on a tawa and cook on both sides with coconut oil, and serve hot.

Other options
Paneer: Tofu, chicken, egg, mixed dal, mixed vegetable, bottle gourd or avocado
For thickening/binding agent, you can use gondu

Serving size (pieces/no)	Energy (Kcal)	Total Carbohydrate (gm)	Fibre (gm)	Fat (gm)	Protein (gm)
2 no	345.8	25.18	106.14	13.802	30.44

Amaranth leaves paratha
Ingredients:
100g amaranth leaves | 1 tbsp butter | 1 tsp ghee | 1 tbsp psyllium husk | 1/4 cup coconut flour| 2 garlic cloves | salt for taste

Preparation method:
1. Heat oil in a pan over a low flame, add amaranth leaves, green chili, garlic, and a pinch of salt.
2. Sauté until tender and grind into a smooth paste.
3. In a bowl, add the coconut flour, psyllium husk, ground paste, salt and warm water. Knead to the consistency of paratha dough.
4. Cover and let the dough rest for 20 minutes.
5. Divide the dough into small balls. Place a dough ball between two pieces of parchment paper and roll into thin, round shape using a rolling pin.
6. Heat a non-stick tawa on medium heat and place the paratha on

it. Smear with ghee and cook for 2 minutes on each side.

7. Serve hot with chutney.

You can add gondu for thickening/binding

Serving size (pieces/no)	Energy (Kcal)	Total Carbohydrate (gm)	Fibre (gm)	Fat (gm)	Protein (gm)
2 no	541.3	35.53	12.05	22.48	19.29

Cauliflower paratha

Ingredients:

100g cauliflower| 1 pinch turmeric | 2 tsp butter | 4 tsp psyllium husk | 3 tbsp coconut flour| 3 tbsp raw almond flour| 1/4 tsp ginger and garlic | 1/4 tsp garam masala powder | 6 tbsp luke warm water | 2 tsp ghee |salt for taste

Preparation method:

1. In a bowl, mix almond flour, coconut flour, psyllium husk, 1 tsp butter, and 1/4 tsp salt. Knead with warm water until it reaches the consistency of a roti dough. Let the dough rest for 10 minutes.

2. For the filling, grate cauliflower and finely chop green chilli.

3. Heat butter in a pan over medium flame, add grated cauliflower, ginger garlic paste, garam masala, green chilli, turmeric powder, and 1/4 tsp salt. Sauté for 2 min.

4. Turn off the heat and add coriander leaves.

5. Separate the dough into four pieces. Place a dough ball between two pieces of parchment paper and roll into a thin, round shape using a rolling pin.

6. Spread half of the filling over one piece of dough. Place another piece of dough on top and gently press the edges together. Repeat with the remaining dough and filling.

7. Heat a non-stick tawa over a medium flame. Place the rolled paratha on it and spread some ghee on the paratha. Cook for 3 minutes on each side.

Other options

Cauliflower: Cabbage, mixed vegetable, paneer, tofu, dal, cheese or egg
You can add psyllium husk or gondu for binding/thickening of the dough.

Serving size (pieces/no)	Energy (Kcal)	Total Carbohydrate (gm)	Fibre (gm)	Fat (gm)	Protein (gm)
2 no	418	32.123	7.573	20.035	12.22

Coconut roti

Ingredients:

1 cup coconut powder (200gm) | 4 tbsp psyllium husk | pinch salt to taste | 1 tbsp curd |2 tbsp buck wheat atta | 2 tbsp butter

Preparation method:

1. Mix all the ingredients with lukewarm water.
2. Keep aside for 30 minutes.
3. Make small balls from the dough. Place a dough ball between two pieces of parchment paper and roll into a thin, round shape using a rolling pin.
4 Heat a tawa on medium flame and place the roti on it.
5. Sprinkle ghee and cook for 2-3 minutes on each side, and serve hot.
Instead of psyllium husk, you can use gondu or xanthan gum

Serving size (pieces/no)	Energy (Kcal)	Total Carbohydrate (gm)	Fibre (gm)	Fat (gm)	Protein (gm)
2 no	295.2	37.66	7.51	10.97	13.04

Flaxseed & groundnut roti

Ingredients:

3 tbsp groundnuts | 1/2 cup flaxseeds | 1/4 cup whole milk | salt for taste | 2 tbsp coconut oil | 2 tbsp grated cheese

Preparation method:

1. In a bowl, mix the powder of flaxseeds and groundnuts with water. Let the batter rest for 20 mins.
2. Mix grated cheese in warm water and add into the batter along with salt. Let the batter be of a thick consistency.
3. Pour the dosa batter on a non-stick pan and sprinkle some oil and cook it on both sides.
Serve it hot with chutney.

Other options

Add psyllium husk or gondu or xanthan gum for binding/thickening of the dough.
Instead of coconut oil, you can use ghee or butter.

Serving size (pieces/no)	Energy (Kcal)	Total Carbohydrate (gm)	Fibre (gm)	Fat (gm)	Protein (gm)
2 no	323	11.09	8.1	28.04	11.73

Coconut cream roti

Ingredients:

1 tsp coconut cream | 1 tbsp ghee | 1 tbsp butter | 1/2 cup coconut flour | 3 tbsp chia seeds | salt to taste

Preparation method:

1. In a bowl, mix coconut flour, chia seed powder, butter, salt, and lukewarm water. Knead to the consistency of a roti dough.
2. Cover and let the dough rest for 15 minutes.
3. Divide the dough into small balls. Place a dough ball between

two pieces of parchment paper and roll into a thin, round shape using a rolling pin.
4. Heat a non-stick tawa on medium heat and place the roti. Smear the roti with ghee and cook for 2 minutes on each side.
Serve the roti warm with chutney.

Serving size (pieces/no)	Energy (Kcal)	Total Carbohydrate (gm)	Fibre (gm)	Fat (gm)	Protein (gm)
2 no	322	48.3	6.3	13.14	10.12

Seeds roti

Ingredients:

2 tbsp chia seeds | 3 tsp coconut oil | 1/4 cup chopped onions | 1 tbsp ginger | 1 tsp cumin | 1 cup sunflower seeds | 2 tbsp sesame seeds | 1/4 cup curd | salt for taste | 2 tsp psyllium husk |1 tsp gondu |1 cup luke warm water

Preparation method:

1. In a bowl, mix sunflower seed flour, sesame seed powder, chia seed powder, chopped onions, curry leaves, green chilli, ginger, salt and cumin seeds.
2. Add lukewarm water and knead to a roti dough consistency. Pat over a butter paper or parchment paper.
3. Spread some oil over the roti and cook on medium flame. Flip over and cook on the other side till done.
Serve it warm with coconut chutney.

Other options

Instead of sunflower seeds and sesame seeds, you can use pumpkin and water melon seeds
Add psyllium husk or gondu for binding/thickening of the dough

Serving size (pieces/no)	Energy (Kcal)	Total Carbohydrate (gm)	Fibre (gm)	Fat (gm)	Protein (gm)
2 no	254.6	15.28	7.15	20.686	8.011

Bottle Gourd Talipattu

Ingredients:

1 cup bottle gourd | 1/4 cup sunflower seeds | 2 tsp ghee |
1/2 tsp xanthan gum| 2 green chillies | 1/4 cup almonds |
1/4 tsp ginger | 1/2 tsp ground dry chilli | 1/2 tsp cumin |
1/2 tsp garam masala | salt to taste| lukewarm water

Preparation method:

1. Grind sunflower seeds and almonds into a fine powder.
2. Grate bottle gourd and squeeze out the water. Finely chop green chilli.
3. In a bowl, mix the ground powder, xanthan gum, bottle gourd, cumin seeds, green chillies, ginger, red chilli powder (optional), garam masala, and salt. Knead to the consistency of a roti dough.
4. Divide the dough into uniform balls. Place a dough ball between two pieces of parchment paper and roll into a thin, round shape using a rolling pin.
5. Heat a non-stick tawa on medium heat and place the talipattu on it. Spread some ghee on the talipattu and cook for 2 minutes on each side.
Serve warm with coconut chutney.

Other options:

Instead of bottle gourd, you can use ridge gourd, cucumber, pumpkin or ash gourd

Serving size (pieces/no)	Energy (Kcal)	Total Carbohydrate (gm)	Fibre (gm)	Fat (gm)	Protein (gm)
2 no	238.9	13.34	9.38	12.342	5.05

Nuts and seeds chapathi

Ingredients:

6 tbsp almonds | 1/2 tbsp chia seeds | 2 tsp ghee | 6 tbsp water melon seeds |1 tsp butter | 1/2 tsp xanthan gum/gondu | salt for taste | 1 cup lukewarm water

Preparation method:

1. Mix all the ingredients in a bowl, knead the flour with luke warm water and make small balls.
2. Take two parchment paper, place the dough in between and roll thinly to round shape.
3. Heat a tawa on medium flame, place the chapathi, spread some ghee and cook on both sides.
Serve hot with mint chutney.

Other options:

Almonds: any other nuts (except cashew & pistachios)
Watermelon seeds: any oily seeds
Chia seeds: basil seeds

Serving size (pieces/no)	Energy (Kcal)	Total Carbohydrate (gm)	Fibre (gm)	Fat (gm)	Protein (gm)
2 no	243.49	13.86	11.919	12.656	3.619

Garlic naan

Ingredients:

6 tbsp coconut flour| 2 tbsp curd | 2 tsp coconut oil | 1/2 tsp xanthan gum | 1 tbsp psyllium husks | 1/2 tsp baking powder | 2 garlic cloves | 1/4 tsp sesame seeds | 1/2 cup luke warm water | salt to taste

Preparation method:

1. In a bowl, add coconut flour, psyllium husk, xanthan gum, baking powder, thick curd, salt, and warm water. Knead to the consistency of a soft dough.
2. Cover and let the dough rest for 20 minutes.
3. Divide the dough into two uniform balls. Place a dough ball between two pieces of parchment paper and roll into an oval shape using a rolling pin.
4. Sprinkle sesame seeds and minced garlic on top of the rolled naan.
5. Heat a non-stick tawa over medium heat and place the naan.

Sprinkle coconut oil and cook for 5 min and serve warm.

Other options

Add psyllium husk or gondu for binding/thickening of the dough
Instead of curd, you can use butter, ghee or cream

Serving size (pieces/no)	Energy (Kcal)	Total Carbohydrate (gm)	Fibre (gm)	Fat (gm)	Protein (gm)
2 no	321.3	36.153	12.6	15.06	10.4

Bhakri

Ingredients:

1/4 cup coconut flour | 1 tbsp psyllium husks | 1 tbsp cheese | 2 tbsp raw almond flour | 1 pinch corn starch | pinch of baking powder | 1 tbsp coconut oil | salt to taste

Preparation method:

1. In a bowl, mix coconut flour, almond flour, psyllium husk, cheese, baking powder, salt and luke warm water. Knead to the consistency of a roti dough.
2. Cover and let the dough rest for 20 minutes.
3. Divide the dough into small balls. Place a dough ball between two pieces of parchment paper and roll into a thin, round shape using a rolling pin.
4. Heat a non-stick tawa on medium heat and place the bhakri. Grease with coconut oil and cook for 2 minutes on each side. Serve warm with kurma.

Other options

Psyllium husk: Gondu for binding/thickening of the dough

Serving size (pieces/no)	Energy (Kcal)	Total Carbohydrate (gm)	Fibre (gm)	Fat (gm)	Protein (gm)
2 no	326.6	29.633	6.173	18.2	12.0

Coconut & cauliflower rice

Ingredients:

1/2 cup shredded coconut | 1/2 cup cauliflower rice | 1/4 tsp mustard seeds | 2 tbsp coconut oil | 5 almonds | 1 dried red chilli | a pinch of hing | salt for taste

Preparation method:

1. Chop almonds into small pieces.
2. Heat oil in a pan and add the mustard seeds.
3. Once the mustard starts popping, add dry red chilli, hing, curry leaves, coconut and almond pieces and sauté.
4. Add cauliflower rice and salt, and mix well.
Serve warm with dal or Sāmbhar.

Other options

Instead of coconut oil: Ghee or butter
Instead of cauliflower: Cabbage or broccoli

Serving size (gm/cup)	Energy (Kcal)	Total Carbohydrate (gm)	Fibre (gm)	Fat (gm)	Protein (gm)
1 cup (100 gm)	108.9	10.9	3.4	7.38	2.66

Cauliflower methi rice

Ingredients:

1/4 tsp salt | 200g cauliflower rice | a pinch of turmeric powder | 2 cloves | 1 ½ tsp ghee | 1/2 tomato | 1/2 onion | 1/2 tsp ginger garlic paste | 1 green chilli |1/2 tsp coriander powder | 1/2 tsp red chilli powder | 1 cardamom | 1 bay leaf | 1/2 tsp cumin powder | 1/4 cup water | 75gm methi (fenugreek) leaves

Preparation method:

1. Grind onion to a smooth paste and finely chop methi leaves,

tomato and green chilli.
2. Grate cauliflower into "rice".
3. Add grated cauliflower to a pan with 2 cups of boiling water. Cover and cook for 2 minutes over medium heat.
4. Drain the grated cauliflower using a colander or muslin cloth and squeeze out the excess water.
5. Warm ghee in a pan over medium heat. Add bay leaf, cardamom, and clove. Add ground onion, ginger garlic paste and green chilli, and sauté until it turns brown.
6. Add chopped tomato, turmeric powder, coriander powder, red chilli powder, cumin powder, salt and water.
7. Lower the heat and add methi leaves. Sauté until soft
8. Add the cauliflower rice and mix well, cover, cook for 3 minutes and serve warm.

Other options

Cauliflower: Cabbage or broccoli

Serving size (gm/cup)	Energy (Kcal)	Total Carbohydrate (gm)	Fibre (gm)	Fat (gm)	Protein (gm)
1 cup (100 gm)	105.9	10.97	3.4	6.88	2.66

Cauliflower palak rice

Ingredients:

1/4 tsp salt | 100g spinach | 200g cauliflower| 2 tbsp ghee | 1/2 cup onion | 2 green chillies | 1/2 tsp cumin seeds | 1 bay leaf| 3 tbsp water | 2 garlic cloves | Salt for taste

Preparation method:

1. Finely chop onion and garlic.
2. Grate the cauliflower into "rice".
3. Add grated cauliflower and ¼ tsp salt to a pan with 2 cups of boiling water. Cover and cook for 2 minutes over medium heat.
4. Drain the grated cauliflower using a colander or muslin cloth and squeeze out the excess water.

5. Warm ghee in a pan over medium flame. Add cumin seeds and bay leaf. After the cumin seeds start to pop, add the onion, garlic, spinach and sauté for a minute.

6. Add the ground paste, remaining salt, cauliflower rice and mix well.

Serve warm.

Other options

Instead of ghee, you can use butter or coconut oil

Serving size (gm/cup)	Energy (Kcal)	Total Carbohydrate (gm)	Fibre (gm)	Fat (gm)	Protein (gm)
1 cup (100 gm)	105.07	10.12	3.1	7.17	2.91

Cauliflower lemon rice

Ingredients:

1 ½ cup cauliflower| 1 pinch turmeric | 1/4 tsp mustard seeds | 1 tbsp coconut oil | 2 green chillies | 4-5 curry leaves |1/4 tsp ginger | 1 tbsp peanuts | 2 tsp lemon juice | 1 pinch hing | salt for taste

Preparation method:

1. Squeeze lemon in cauliflower rice and add salt as required.
2. Heat pan with oil and add mustard.
3. Once mustard starts popping, add green chilli, hing, curry leaves, turmeric powder and ginger.
4. Then add tempering to the cauliflower lemon rice and mix well and serve hot.

Other options

Instead of coconut oil, you can use ghee or butter. You can also use cumin seeds for the seasoning.

Serving size (gm/cup)	Energy (Kcal)	Total Carbohydrate (gm)	Fibre (gm)	Fat (gm)	Protein (gm)
1 cup (100 gm)	129.7	5.04	2.676	77.3	3.75

Cauliflower bisi bele bath

Ingredients:

3 tbsp grated coconut | 1 cup cauliflower rice| 1/4 tsp turmeric | 1/4 tsp mustard seeds | 3 tbsp ghee | 1 cinnamon stick | 2 green beans | 4 almonds | 1 tsp lemon juice | 1 tsp cumin | 1 tsp poppy seed | 1/4 tsp hing | 5 tbsp coriander seeds |1/2 tsp fenugreek | salt to taste| other vegetables| curry leaves| red chilly

Preparation method:

1. Dry roast coriander seeds, fenugreek, cumin, poppy seed, cinnamon stick, asafoetida and grated coconut one by one. Grind into a fine powder.
2. Cut all the vegetables in 1/2-inch size. Heat ghee in a pan, add all vegetables and sauté for 2 minutes.
3. Add 1/2 cup water, salt and cook the vegetables. Now add cauliflower rice, turmeric powder and grounded masala powder.
4. Cover and cook in low flame till it reaches a thick consistency. Now add lemon juice and mix well.
5. Tempering - Heat ghee in a pan, add mustard seeds, allow it to pop and add chopped almonds, dry red chilli and curry leaves.
6. Add the above tempering to the Bisi bele bath, garnish with coriander leaves and serve hot.

Other options

Garnish: Dry coconut flakes, sesame seeds, fresh coconut flakes
Instead of cauliflower rice, you can use cabbage or broccoli rice

Serving size (gm/cup)	Energy (Kcal)	Total Carbohydrate (gm)	Fibre (gm)	Fat (gm)	Protein (gm)
1 cup (100 gm)	184.2	13.66	5.5	13.3	5.136

Cauliflower curd rice

Ingredients:

1/2 cup whole milk plain curd |1 cup cauliflower rice| 1/4 tsp mustard seeds | 1/4 tbsp coconut oil | 1 pinch hing | salt to taste| green chilly| curry leaves

Preparation method:

1. In a bowl, add cauliflower rice, curd, green chilli and salt as required.
2. Heat oil in a pan and add mustard seeds.
3. Once mustard starts popping, add curry leaves and hing.
4. Add tempering to the cauliflower curd rice.
Garnish the curd rice with coriander leaves and serve.

Other options

Instead of coconut oil: Ghee or butter
Instead of cauliflower rice: Cabbage or broccoli rice
Instead of normal curd: Plant based curd
Add green gram dal or urad dal for seasoning

Serving size (gm/cup)	Energy (Kcal)	Total Carbohydrate (gm)	Fibre (gm)	Fat (gm)	Protein (gm)
1 cup (100 gm)	86.17	4.5	1.6	6.79	2.2

Cauliflower fried rice

Ingredients:

1 tsp apple cider vinegar | 1 cup cauliflower| 1/2 bell peppers | 4 green beans | 1 tbsp coconut oil | 2 tbsp chopped onions | 1/2 tsp ginger | 1/2 tsp pepper | 2 garlic cloves | Salt to taste

Preparation method:

1.Grate the cauliflower into rice
2. Heat oil in a pan.
3. Add chopped garlic and ginger and sauté till they are slightly done.
4. Add remaining chopped vegetables and fry for 2-3 mins until vegetables are cooked.
5. Finally add cauliflower rice, vinegar, pepper powder and salt as required. Mix everything well and sauté for 2 mins, and serve hot.

Other options

Sauce: Chilli sauce, soya sauce
Garnish: Coriander leaves or spring onions
Instead of cauliflower rice use cabbage or broccoli rice

Serving size (gm/cup)	Energy (Kcal)	Total Carbohydrate (gm)	Fibre (gm)	Fat (gm)	Protein (gm)
1 cup (100 gm)	115.8	12.31	3.822	6.44	3.72

Cauliflower poha

Ingredients:

1 cup cauliflower| 1 pinch turmeric | 1/4 tsp mustard seeds | 1 ½ tbsp ghee | 2 tbsp peanuts| 1 onion | 2 green chilli | 1 tbsp coriander leaves | 2 tsp lemon juice | 1 tbsp curry leaves |1 tbsp coconut oil | salt to taste

Preparation method:

1. Separate the cauliflower florets and stalks.
2. Cut the stalks into cubes (similar to potato cubes).
3. Boil the stalks in salted water till tender. Keep them aside in a bowl.
4. Grate the florets and cook them in boiling water with salt. Drain and squeeze out the water.
5. Heat ghee in a pan on medium flame. Fry the peanuts and keep aside.
6. Add mustard seeds and once they start popping, add onions, green chillies, curry leaves and turmeric powder. Sauté for 2 minutes.
7. Add the boiled cauliflower rice, cauliflower stalks and mix well.
8. Garnish with coriander leaves and add lemon juice, and serve warm.

Serving size (gm/cup)	Energy (Kcal)	Total Carbohydrate (gm)	Fibre (gm)	Fat (gm)	Protein (gm)
1 cup (100 gm)	193.3	9.63	3.8	16.6	4.8

Pumpkin pulao

Ingredients:

2 cups grated pumpkin | 2 tbsp beans | 2 tbsp peas | 1 cup cauliflower| 2 tsp mint leaves |2 tsp coriander leaves | 1 cup onions | 2 tbsp coconut oil | 2 green chillies | salt to taste| 2 green chillies|1 tsp chilli powder |1 tsp garam masala powder

Preparation method:

1. Cut beans, cauliflower and onions in desired shape.
2. Boil the vegetables with little salt, chilli powder and garam masala. Keep it aside.
3. Heat coconut oil in a pan. Add finely chopped onions and sauté for 2 minutes.
4. Add green chillies and mint leaves and fry for 2 minutes.

5. Add grated pumpkin and fry on medium heat, till it becomes soft.

6. Add the cooked vegetables and mix it nicely. Add salt to taste.

7. Garnish with coriander leaves and serve hot.

Other options

Pumpkin: Ash gourd or squash
Cauliflower rice: Cabbage or broccoli rice
Coconut oil: Ghee or butter
Add hing for digestion

Serving size (gm/cup)	Energy (Kcal)	Total Carbohydrate (gm)	Fibre (gm)	Fat (gm)	Protein (gm)
1 cup (100 gm)	125	17.52	4.8	5.94	4.304

Vegetable khichdi

Ingredients:

2 cup cauliflower| one pinch turmeric | pinch of mustard seeds | 1 tsp butter | 1/4 tsp xanthan gum | 2 green beans | 2 dried red chilli | 1/4 tsp ground dry chilli | 1/2 tsp cumin| pinch hing powder |1/2 tsp mixed spices (biryani masala) | 2 tsp flaxseed | 5gm almonds | ½ cup chironji seeds (charoli nuts) | salt for taste

Preparation method:

1. Soak chironji seeds in 1/2 cup of water for 1 hour. Grind it coarsely without adding water.

2. Grate the cauliflower into "rice".

3. In a pressure cooker, cook the grated cauliflower, ground chironji, beans, flaxseeds powder, turmeric powder, chilli powder, biryani masala and water for 3 whistles.

4. Warm ghee in a pan over medium flame. Once warm, add mustard seeds and let it splutter. Add cumin seeds, asafoetida, cooked cauliflower rice mix, salt and xanthan gum. Cook on low heat for 3 minutes, and serve warm.

Other options

Chironji seeds: Green gram dal, toor dal or chana dal
Cauliflower rice: Cabbage or broccoli rice
Butter: Coconut oil or ghee

Serving size (gm/cup)	Energy (Kcal)	Total Carbohydrate (gm)	Fibre (gm)	Fat (gm)	Protein (gm)
1 cup (100 gm)	156.9	12.33	5.876	10.5	5.0

Baked veg au gratin

Ingredients:

1 ½ cup cauliflower| 1/4 cup mushroom | 1/4 avocado | 3 slices of cheese | 1 tbsp red chilli powder | 1/2 tbsp jeera powder | 1/2 tbsp coriander powder | salt to taste | 1 tbsp mixed herbs | 1 tbsp butter/ghee

Preparation method:

1. Melt ghee/butter in a stir fry pan and sauté the vegetables with salt.
2. Add all the spice powders and half cook the vegetables to retain their crunchiness
4. Transfer the vegetables to a microwave & OTG safe tin.
5. Add 2-3 tbsp of tomato sauce and mix well.
6. Layer the top with shredded cheese/ cheese slice.
7. Sprinkle mixed herbs.
8. Bake it at 160° C for 10 minutes or microwave it until cheese melts.

Serving size (gm/cup)	Energy (Kcal)	Total Carbohydrate (gm)	Fibre (gm)	Fat (gm)	Protein (gm)
1 cup (100 gm)	177.97	6.5	3.7	15.18	6.75

Kadhi

250ml full fat yogurt | 1/4 cup gram flour| 20gm ginger chilli paste |1/4 tsp fenugreek seeds| 1/4 tsp cumin | 1/4 tsp fennel seeds | 1/4 tsp mustard | 1 dried red chilli| 3 tbsp ghee | 1/4 cup coriander leaves | pinch of hing |750ml water | 1/4 tsp turmeric | 1/4 salt to taste | red chilli powder to taste.

1. In a bowl, mix the yogurt, gram flour, and water using a hand blender.
2. Place the yogurt-flour-water mixture in a pot and place it on a medium flame.
3. Once the mixture gets warm, add the ginger chilli paste. Keep stirring continuously or the mixture will split.
4. Add coriander leaves, curry leaves and salt.
5. Bring the kadhi to a boil and reduce the heat setting. Let it simmer for another 10-15 minutes. Continue stirring to prevent curdling.
6. Tempering – Warm ghee in a saucepan and add dry red chilli, whole spices and stir frequently.
7. Once the spices start releasing aroma, add red chilli powder, turmeric and asafoetida.
8. Add the tempering and simmer the kadhi for about 15 min.
9. If it's too thick, add more water. Add salt according to taste.
10. Garnish with chopped coriander leaves and serve hot.

Serving size (ml/cup)	Energy (Kcal)	Total Carbohydrate (gm)	Fibre (gm)	Fat (gm)	Protein (gm)
1 cup (100 ml)	140.3	9.25	2.47	8.3	8.45

BAKERY

Peanut Butter Balls

Ingredients:

2 cups cream cheese | 1/2 cup unsweetened peanut butter | 1/4 cup coconut oil | pinch salt |1/2 cup dark chocolate chips

Preparation method:

1. Line a parchment paper in a bowl.
2. Combine the cream cheese, peanut butter, ¼ cup coconut oil, and salt.
3. Beat the mixture for about 2 minutes until fully combined. Place the bowl in the freezer for 10-15 minutes to firm up slightly.
4. When the peanut butter mixture has hardened, use a small cookie scoop to create tablespoon-sized balls. Place it in the refrigerator to harden, for about 5 minutes.
5. To make the chocolate drizzle: combine the chocolate chips and coconut oil, in a microwave safe bowl and microwave in 30 second intervals until fully melted.
6. Drizzle it over the peanut butter balls and place them back in the refrigerator to harden, for about 5 minutes.
7. Store peanut butter balls in the refrigerator.

Serving size (pieces/no)	Energy (Kcal)	Total Carbohydrate (gm)	Fibre (gm)	Fat (gm)	Protein (gm)
2 no	413	10.61	2	36.7	13.61

Laddu

Ingredients:

¼ cup grated coconut | 25gm almonds | ¼ tsp sesame seeds | 1 tbsp ghee | 1 tsp pumpkin seeds | ¼ cup watermelon seeds | 2 tbsp stevia | pinch of cardamom powder

Preparation method:

1. Heat a pan over medium heat. Dry roast almonds and melon seeds. Grind into a fine powder.
2. In a bowl, mix the ground powder, cardamom powder, and stevia.
3. Grind the pumpkin seeds coarsely.
4. Heat ghee in a pan on medium heat, add pumpkin seeds, coconut and white sesame seeds.
5. Turn off the heat and add to dry mixture and stir to combine.
6. Make small balls from the mixture to form laddus.

Serving size (pieces/no)	Energy (Kcal)	Total Carbohydrate (gm)	Fibre (gm)	Fat (gm)	Protein (gm)
1 no	380	20.1	5.3	6	6.5

Jamun

Ingredients:

2 tbsp coconut flour| 3 tbsp almond flour | ¼ cup stevia | ¼ cup water | ½ tsp cardamom powder | pinch of baking powder | 2 tbsp coconut oil | ½ tsp xanthan gum | ½ cup cheese

Preparation method:

1. In a bowl, mix cheese, almond flour, coconut flour, xanthan gum, baking powder and knead to the consistency of a soft dough.
2. Divide the dough into small balls and let it rest for 5 minutes. (Do not keep the dough for long duration).
3. To make the syrup in a pan, bring water to boil on medium heat. Add stevia and cardamom powder. Cook for 5 minutes and turn off the heat.
4. Heat coconut oil in a pan over medium heat. Once warm, add jamun balls. Fry on all sides until golden.
5. Add fried jamun in the warm stevia syrup and serve warm or cold.

Serving size (pieces/no)	Energy (Kcal)	Total Carbohydrate (gm)	Fibre (gm)	Fat (gm)	Protein (gm)
2 no	679	19.5	9	58.9	21

Pumpkin Cheese Balls
Ingredients:
4 tsp coconut flour| 4 tsp almond flour| 300 gm pumpkin | 40 gm cheddar cheese | ¼ tsp black pepper | pinch of salt

Preparation method:
1. Peel the pumpkin skin and cut into small pieces.
2. Pressure cook pumpkin with ½ cup water for 2 whistles.
3. After the pressure settles down, drain the boiled pumpkin and mash into smooth paste.
4. Heat an empty pan on high heat, add mashed pumpkin and sauté to remove excess moisture. Allow the mashed pumpkin to cool.
5. In a bowl, mix mashed pumpkin, coconut flour, almond flour, black pepper powder, and salt. Knead the dough to a soft consistency.
6. Cut the cheese into small cubes and place the cheese inside the pumpkin dough. Make round balls like these and set aside.
7. Heat coconut oil in a pan over medium heat. Once warm, lower the flame and add the cheese balls.
8. Fry until golden and serve warm.

Other options
Pumpkin paneer balls

Serving size (pieces/no)	Energy (Kcal)	Total Carbohydrate (gm)	Fibre (gm)	Fat (gm)	Protein (gm)
4 no	244.51	9.89	3.842	37.9	6.3

Flax Seed Bread
Ingredients:

3 cups almond flour| 1/2 cup flaxseeds | ½ tbsp baking powder | 1 tsp sea salt | 4 eggs | ½ cup unsalted butter | 1 cup warm water

Preparation method:

1. Preheat the oven to 350°F (177°C), line a loaf pan with parchment paper.
2. In a large bowl, stir together almond flour, flaxseed meal, baking powder, and sea salt.
3. Stir eggs and melted butter, then stir with warm water.
4. Mix well until air bubbles appear and then add flaxseeds.
5. Transfer the batter to the lined baking pan. Smoothen the top evenly to form a rounded surface. Sprinkle more flaxseeds over the top, if desired.
6. Bake for 45-50 minutes to get a crusty, brown top.

Other options

Eggless bread, almond bun

Serving size (pieces/no)	Energy (Kcal)	Total Carbohydrate (gm)	Fibre (gm)	Fat (gm)	Protein (gm)
2 slices	1540.7	53.27	38.85	134.75	50.05

Multi Seeds Bread
Ingredients:

¼ cup unsalted sunflower seeds | ¼ cup unsalted pumpkin seeds | 3 tbsp flaxseeds | 3 tbsp sesame seeds | 1 ¾ cup almond flour| ¼ cup coconut flour| 1 tbsp baking powder | ¼ tsp salt | 3 large eggs | 1 cup buttermilk | ¼ cup coconut oil | 1 tbsp chia seeds | 1 tbsp stevia drops

Preparation method:

1. Preheat an oven to 350° F. Line the bottom of a loaf pan with parchment paper.

2. In a pan, dry roast sunflower seeds, pumpkin seeds, flaxseeds and sesame seeds over medium heat, until it turns light brown.
3. Reserve 2 tablespoons of the seed mixture in a small bowl; transfer the remaining seeds to a large bowl.
4. In a bowl, add the roasted seeds, almond flour, coconut flour, baking powder, baking soda and salt.
5. Whisk eggs, buttermilk, oil, chia seeds and stevia drops in another bowl. Stir all the ingredients until combined well.
6. Transfer the batter to the lined baking pan. Smooth the top evenly, sprinkle the reserved seeds, pressing them gently into the batter to help them adhere. Let stand for 10 minutes.
7. Bake until golden brown for about 40 minutes. Cool the pan for 30 minutes.
8. Remove from the pan when completely cooled.
9. Multi seeds bread is now ready to eat.

Other options
Eggless bread, almond bun

Serving size (pieces/no)	Energy (Kcal)	Total Carbohydrate (gm)	Fibre (gm)	Fat (gm)	Protein (gm)
2 slices	884.1	34.65	16.17	74.9	31.15

Low Carb Bread/Bun
Ingredients:
7 eggs | 2 cups almond flour| ½ cup unsalted butter | 2 tbsp chia seeds | 3 tbsp sesame seeds | 1 tsp baking powder | ½ tsp xanthan gum

Preparation method:
1. Preheat oven to 180°C (355°F)
2. In a mixing bowl, whisk the eggs together.
3. Add the remaining ingredients and mix well. Using an electric whisk or hand mixer can make the mixture thick.
4. Pour into a loaf pan lined with baking paper. Place sesame seeds on top.
5. Bake for 40 minutes and cool completely before removing from

the pan.

6. Low carb bread is now ready to eat.

7. Best kept in the fridge for up to 5 days, or frozen for up to 3 weeks.

Other options

Eggless bread, almond bun, flaxseeds bread, multi seeds bread

Serving size (pieces/no)	Energy (Kcal)	Total Carbohydrate (gm)	Fibre (gm)	Fat (gm)	Protein (gm)
2 slices	609.7	14.805	21.608	52.82	26.06

2 Minute Instant Bread

Ingredients:

¼ cup Almond flour | 1 tbsp coconut flour | 1 tbsp unsalted butter | 1/8 tsp baking powder | 1 egg

Preparation method:

1. Place all the ingredients in a mug and combine them well.

2. Microwave it only for 90 seconds.

3. Let it cool down.

4. Loosen the bread from the edges of the mug using a knife.

5. Flip the mug upside down, and slice the bread.

Other options

Pumpkin bread, zucchini bread, sesame seed bread

Serving size (pieces/no)	Energy (Kcal)	Total Carbohydrate (gm)	Fibre (gm)	Fat (gm)	Protein (gm)
2 slices	501	14.87	5.9	43.65	12.73

Keto egg bread

Ingredients:

250 gm cheese | 8 eggs | 50 gm butter| 1 tbsp stevia | 1 tbsp cold water | 1 tbsp gelatin powder | 1 tbsp hot water | 1 tsp cinnamon powder | ¼ tsp nut meg

Preparation method:

1. Preheat the oven to 180°C (355°F).
2. In a mixing bowl, beat the cream cheese with eggs, butter, and stevia until it becomes a smooth paste.
3. Combine cold water and gelatin powder to rehydrate the gelatin. Leave it to sit for 3 minutes.
4. Remove gelatin from cold water and transfer to hot water, then beat into the egg mixture.
5. Line a loaf pan with baking paper and pour the batter into the tin.
6. Sprinkle with cinnamon and nutmeg, and gently stir it in with a spoon. This will give the loaf a brown colour on top.
7. Cook in the oven for 40 minutes and cool completely before removing from the pan.
8. Keto egg bread is now ready to eat.

Other options

Keto naan bread, low carb sesame crisp bread, low carb poppy seed bread, nut free bread

Serving size (pieces/no)	Energy (Kcal)	Total Carbohydrate (gm)	Fibre (gm)	Fat (gm)	Protein (gm)
2 slices	337.25	2.85	0.708	27.04	22.07

Low carb granola bars

Ingredients:

9 tbsp almonds | 2 tbsp walnuts | 6 tbsp sesame seeds | 7 tbsp pumpkin seeds | 2 tbsp flaxseeds | 2/3 cup shredded coconut | dark chocolate | 6 tbsp coconut oil | 4 tbsp sesame paste | 1 tsp vanilla paste | 2 tsp ground cinnamon | pinch salt

Preparation method:

1. Preheat the oven to 350°F (175°C).
2. Mix all the ingredients in a blender or food processor to get a coarse mixture.
3. Spoon the mixture into a baking dish, preferably lined with parchment paper.
4. Bake for 15–20 minutes, or until the mixture turns golden brown.
5. Let it cool before removing from the baking dish. Divide into pieces with a sharp knife.
6. Melt the chocolate using a double boiler or microwave oven.
7. Top the granola bars with melted chocolate.

Other options

Nuts granola, nuts bar, almond butter bars

Serving size (pieces/no)	Energy (Kcal)	Total Carbohydrate (gm)	Fibre (gm)	Fat (gm)	Protein (gm)
1 no	365.21	13.07	5.47	31.93	10.426

Peanut butter cookies

Ingredients:

¾ cup peanut butter | 2/3 cup stevia | 1 egg | ½ tsp vanilla extract | ½ salt | ¼ cup butter.

Preparation method:

1. Preheat oven to 360°F (180°C). Make sure the butter is soft, and mix all the ingredients in a bowl until well combined.
2. Roll them into small balls and squash flat with a fork.
3. Bake for 15 – 20 mins until slightly brown.
4. Cool on a baking tray for 20 mins and enjoy!

Other options

Eggless almond cookies, coconut cookies, peanut cookies, nut cookies

Serving size (pieces/no)	Energy (Kcal)	Total Carbohydrate (gm)	Fibre (gm)	Fat (gm)	Protein (gm)
1 no	335.6	8.1	1.8	30.5	11.8

Lemon coconut cake

Ingredients:

½ cup coconut flour | 5 eggs | ½ cup stevia | ½ cup butter | ½ lemon | ½ tsp lemon zest | ½ tsp xanthan gum | ½ tsp salt | 1 cup cream cheese | 3 tbsp stevia | 1 tsp vanilla extract | ½ tsp lemon zest

Preparation method:

1. Separate the egg whites and yolks. Beat the egg whites until they form white peaks.
2. Add the remaining ingredients to the same bowl and combine well.
3. Pour into a greased loaf pan.
4. Bake at 180° C (355°F) for 45 mins.
5. While the cake is in the oven, beat the cream cheese, stevia, vanilla extract and lemon zest together with an electric beater or hand beater.
7. Set aside and let the cake cool down
8. Ice the cake
Lemon coconut cake is now ready to eat

Other options

Almond flour brownie, almond cake, almond flour muffins, chocolate muffins with almond flour

Serving size (pieces/no)	Energy (Kcal)	Total Carbohydrate (gm)	Fibre (gm)	Fat (gm)	Protein (gm)
1 no	284.6	11.04	5.08	24.64	8.3

Brownie bites

Ingredients:

¼ cup creamy almond butter | ¼ cup stevia drops | ¼ cup chocolate chips | 2 tbsp almond flour| 3 tbsp cocoa powder | 1 pinch salt

Preparation method:

1. Add all wet ingredients into a medium microwave safe bowl. Melt for about 40 to 60 seconds. Remove from microwave and stir well, until chocolate chips melt and becomes a smooth mixture.
2. Add all dry ingredients to the wet ingredients and stir well to make a smooth dough.
3. Roll dough into small bite size balls (if dough feels too soft or sticky to work with, then leave aside at room temperature for a few minutes to thicken and firm up).
4. Let bites cool completely (they will continue to firm up even more as it cools) before storing in an air tight container.

Serving size (pieces/no)	Energy (Kcal)	Total Carbohydrate (gm)	Fibre (gm)	Fat (gm)	Protein (gm)
1 no	571.9	38.5	10.85	44.45	16.59

SNACKS

Ladies finger fry

Ingredients:

¼ cup sunflower seeds | 1 tbsp sesame seeds | 1/4 tsp turmeric powder | 200gm ladies finger| 4 tbsp coconut oil | ¼ tsp ginger | ½ tsp garam masala powder | ¾ tsp coriander powder | ¾ tsp red chilli powder | 1 tsp lemon juice | ¼ tsp cumin powder

Preparation method:

1. Roast sunflower seeds, sesame seeds and grind into a fine powder. Add chilli powder, turmeric, coriander powder, cumin powder, garam masala, ginger paste, and salt in a bowl and mix well. Add lemon juice to the mixture.
2. Cut the ladies finger into two halves and sideways and mix with the spice's mixture.
3. Marinate for 10 minutes.
4. Heat a pan, pour oil and deep fry the marinated ladies finger on medium flame till they turn crispy.
5. Serve hot.

Other options

Avocado chips, baked zucchini chips

Serving size (pieces/no)	Energy (Kcal)	Total Carbohydrate (gm)	Fibre (gm)	Fat (gm)	Protein (gm)
4 no	244.51	9.89	3.842	37.9	6.3

Avocado chips

Ingredients:

1 tsp lime juice | ½ cup avocado | ½ tsp garlic powder | ½ tsp onion powder | ½ tsp oregano | salt for taste

Preparation method:

1. Preheat the oven to 325° F and line a baking pan with parchment paper.
2. Add all the ingredients in a bowl and mix until you get a smooth batter.
3. Scoop the mixture on the lined pan, leaving 2 - 3 inches of space in between the scoops.
4. Using your fingers or the back of a spoon to press down each of the scoops into a 3-inch-wide circle.
5. Place the baking pan in the oven, and bake it for about 35- 40 minutes or until the chips turn crispy.
6. Remove the chips from the oven. Place them on a cooling rack and let them cool down completely.
7. Serve with your favourite dip and enjoy.

Serving size (pieces/no)	Energy (Kcal)	Total Carbohydrate (gm)	Fibre (gm)	Fat (gm)	Protein (gm)
4 no	244.51	9.89	3.842	37.9	6.3

Low carb veg samosa
Ingredients:

1 tsp butter | 1 cup cauliflower| 4 tbsp onion | 1 tbsp ginger paste | ½ tsp coriander seeds powder | 1 tsp garam masala | ¼ tsp cumin seeds | ¼ tsp red chilli flakes| ¾ cup almond flour| ½ cup mozzarella cheese

Preparation method:
For the filling:
1. Preheat a pan over medium heat, add butter, onions and cauliflower.
2. Sprinkle salt over the vegetables. Cook by stirring occasionally until the vegetables are cooked.
3. Add ginger paste, coriander, garam masala, ground cumin seeds and chilli flakes. Stir for 1-2 minutes and turn off the heat.
4. Preheat oven to 375° F.

For the dough:

1. Set up a double boiler. Use a large sauce pan with about 1 ½ - 2 inch of water in it and a medium mixing bowl that fits on top.
2. Bring the water in the lower part of the double boiler to a simmer over high heat. Once it is simmering turn heat to low.
3. Meanwhile, place the almond flour, cumin, salt and mozzarella in the top part of the double boiler, stir together.
4. Place the bowl containing the almond flour mixture over the simmering water.
5. Stir the mixture constantly until the mozzarella cheese melts and the mixture forms a dough.
6. Place the dough on a parchment paper and knead well.
7. Take small ball size dough, roll the dough into rectangular shape and cut into 2 squares.
8. Fill the centre of each square with the filling. Join the two ends to form a triangle and pinch the edges closed.
9. Place the samosa on the sheet.
10. Fry it until it turns golden and crispy.

Other options

Chicken samosa, egg samosa

Serving size (pieces/no)	Energy (Kcal)	Total Carbohydrate (gm)	Fibre (gm)	Fat (gm)	Protein (gm)
1 no	154.32	11.2	2.816	10.15	7.14

Almond bread cheese sandwich

Ingredients:

1/2 tbsp unsalted butter | 1 slice cheddar cheese | 2 slices almond bread

Preparation method:

1. Heat a pan on medium heat. Add butter to the hot pan, place both slices of bread into the hot butter. Flip the bread and toast on both sides.
2. Place cheese on one side of the bread and place the other bread slice over the cheese.

3. Toast for another minute on both sides until the cheese melts
4. Serve hot.

Other options
Almond bread egg sandwich, almond bread non-veg sandwich

Serving size (pieces/no)	Energy (Kcal)	Total Carbohydrate (gm)	Fibre (gm)	Fat (gm)	Protein (gm)
2 no	519.5	8.4	5.1	43.4	25.28

Cabbage rolls
Ingredients:
450 gm cabbage | 200 gm cauliflower| 60 gm butter | 1 onion | salt to taste | 30 gm heavy whipping cream | ½ tsp ground black pepper | 1 cup coconut milk | 1 tsp soy sauce

Preparation method:
1. Set the oven to 400°F.
2. Remove the root of the cabbage and boil its leaves in slightly salted water for about 3 to 5 minutes. Turn off the heat and let the leaves loosen up.
3. Place a saucepan over medium heat and add butter. Sauté onion and cauliflower in it. Add salt and pepper as per your taste and allow it to cool.
4. Remove the cauliflower–onion mixture in a bowl and add the heavy whipping cream to it. Pour a chunk of this mixture in the middle of each cabbage leaf, fold around the edges, and make a roll.
5. In the same saucepan, sauté the rolls on both sides until the rolls turn slightly brown.
6. Place the cabbage rolls in a microwave-safe bowl or dish and bake for about 30 minutes.
7. Set aside the cabbage juice for the gravy.
8. In a skillet or saucepan, add heavy whipping cream, soy sauce, salt, pepper, and cabbage juice. Bring the mixture to a boil for 5 minutes or until it thickens.

9. Serve the keto cabbage rolls with the gravy.

Serving size (pieces/no)	Energy (Kcal)	Total Carbohydrate (gm)	Fibre (gm)	Fat (gm)	Protein (gm)
1 no	1174	51	14.8	109.4	17.1

Kulfi

Ingredients:

¼ cup almonds | 5 saffron threads | ¼ cup fresh cream | ¼ cup stevia | ¼ cup water

Preparation method:

1. Soak almonds in water for half an hour. Peel the skin and grind it to a smooth paste.
2. Heat a pan over low flame and boil water in it. Once it starts to boil, add fresh cream, stevia and almond paste.
3. Stir continuously until the mixture thickens.
4. Turn off the heat and add saffron strands.
5. Pour the mixture into kulfi moulds and freeze for at least 6 hours.
6. Serve cold.

Serving size (pieces/no)	Energy (Kcal)	Total Carbohydrate (gm)	Fibre (gm)	Fat (gm)	Protein (gm)
1 no	40.8	8.8	3.8	39	8.9

Strawberry ice- cream

Ingredients:

16 oz strawberries | 2 cups heavy cream | 1 teaspoon erythritol

Preparation method:

1. Add strawberries to a blender or food processor and blend until chunky.
2. Set aside 1/4 of the strawberries.

3. Add heavy cream and erythritol to the blender and blend until cream starts to thicken.
4. Add the remaining strawberries and blend it smooth.
5. Pour mixture into a large bowl, cover and freeze for 4-5 hours.
6. Serve and enjoy.

Other options

Butter pecan ice-cream

Serving size (pieces/no)	Energy (Kcal)	Total Carbohydrate (gm)	Fibre (gm)	Fat (gm)	Protein (gm)
1 scoop	141.2	3.872	0.728	13.872	1.36

Non-veg cutlet
Ingredients:

1 egg | ½ tsp salt | 100 gm ground chicken | 200 gm cauliflower| ¼ tsp turmeric powder | ¼ cup coconut oil | 10 almonds | ¼ tsp ginger garlic paste | 2 green chillies | 1 tsp garam masala powder | ¼ tsp black pepper

Preparation method:

1. Chop cauliflower and cook with water for 2 minutes. Coarsely grind the cauliflower.
2. Squeeze out excess water from grounded cauliflower using cotton cloth.
3. Pressure cook the chicken with salt and turmeric powder for 3 whistles. Remove the lid and sauté the chicken until it becomes dry.
4. Grind almonds and green chilli to make a fine paste.
5. In a bowl, beat an egg with crushed pepper and a pinch of salt
6. Knead grounded cauliflower and chicken, almond and green chilli paste, garam masala, ginger garlic paste, salt, half beaten egg into small balls.
7. Flatten the balls to make flat cutlets, brush the cutlet on both sides with the remaining beaten egg paste.
8. Heat coconut oil in a pan over low flame and shallow fry the cutlet on both sides.

9. Serve warm.

Serving size (pieces/no)	Energy (Kcal)	Total Carbohydrate (gm)	Fibre (gm)	Fat (gm)	Protein (gm)
1 no	106.75	1.05	0.375	9.7	4.15

Veg Cutlet

Ingredients:

6 tbsp melted ghee| 1 1/2 teaspoons pepper powder | 500 gms cabbage (medium-sized, coarsely grated) | 1 tsp ginger powder | 1/2 tsp red chilli powder | 1/4 tsp garam masala | 3 tbsp powdered almonds or almond flour | a pinch of turmeric powder | Black pepper | freshly cut coriander

Preparation method:

1. Shred the cabbage and remove the excess water from it and keep it in a bowl. Heat a pan and add 2 tablespoons of ghee to it.
2. Once the ghee is completely melted, sauté garlic, ginger powder and salt. Once the garlic turns brown remove the frying pan from the heat.
3. Add this seasoning to the coarsely grated cabbage and mix thoroughly.
4. Add red chilli powder, garam masala, turmeric powder and pepper powder to the above mixture.
5. Add powdered almonds to the cabbage mixture for thickening it and mix thoroughly.
6. Place a frying pan on low flame and add 5 tablespoons of ghee to it.
7. Take about 1 tablespoon of the cutlet mixture in your hand, shape it into a cutlet. Shape the entire mixture into cutlets and keep it ready.
8. Shallow fry the cutlets on both sides. Do not cook the cutlets on high heat as they will burn and remain raw inside.
9. Serve the cutlets with home-made mint sauce.

Serving size (pieces/no)	Energy (Kcal)	Total Carbohydrate (gm)	Fibre (gm)	Fat (gm)	Protein (gm)
1 no	82.38	2.86	1.06	7.4	1.9

Besan Sev

Ingredients:

¾ cup pumpkin seeds powder | ½ tsp cumin seeds | ¾ tsp xanthan gum | 1 tbsp coconut oil | pinch of Hing (asafoetida) | ½ tsp black pepper | 1.5 tbsp water

Preparation method:

1. Sieve the pumpkin seed powder and crush black pepper coarsely.
2. In a bowl, mix pumpkin seed powder, xanthan gum, cumin seeds, crushed black pepper, asafoetida and salt. Knead with water to a dough consistency.
3. Heat coconut oil in a pan on medium heat, once warm lower the flame.
4. Add the dough to a sev press. Press the dough directly into the pan.
5. Fry until golden and crispy.

Serving size (gm/cup)	Energy (Kcal)	Total Carbohydrate (gm)	Fibre (gm)	Fat (gm)	Protein (gm)
100 gm	355	30.7	9.3	22.5	9.2

Seeds mixture

Ingredients:

3 tbsp sunflower seeds | 2 tbsp sesame seeds | 1 tbsp coconut oil | 3 tbsp pumpkin seeds | 20 almonds | 1 tsp red chilli powder | 1 tsp curry leaves | pinch asafoetida | 1 tbsp desiccated coconut |coriander| salt for taste

Preparation method:

1. Heat a pan on medium flame and add coconut oil. Add hing and curry leaves.
2. Add the sunflower seeds, sesame seeds, pumpkin seeds, and almonds.
3. Roast them well for 2-3 min on low heat.
4. Add red chilli powder, salt, desiccated coconut and chopped coriander and mix well.
5. The seeds mixture is ready to serve.

Serving size (gm/cup)	Energy (Kcal)	Total Carbohydrate (gm)	Fibre (gm)	Fat (gm)	Protein (gm)
100 gm	226	10.2	4.35	19.45	5.45

Chakli

Ingredients:

1 pinch salt | 1/4 cup sunflower seeds | 1/4 tsp sesame seeds | 2 tbsp coconut oil | 2 tbsp roasted peanuts | 1 tbsp besan flour| 2 tbsp water

Preparation method:

1. Grind the sunflower seeds and roasted peanuts into a fine powder.
2. Sieve the sunflower seed, peanut powder and besan into a bowl.
3. Add white sesame seeds, salt and mix well.
4. Mix with water to create a smooth dough.
5. Heat coconut oil in a pan over medium heat.
6. Add the dough inside a chakli press. Press the dough directly into the oil in the pan.
7. Fry both sides until golden.

Serving size (pieces/no)	Energy (Kcal)	Total Carbohydrate (gm)	Fibre (gm)	Fat (gm)	Protein (gm)
4 small pieces	551	12.3	5.1	52.8	12

Vada

Ingredients:

20 gm almonds | ¼ cup onion | ½ tsp red chilli powder | 2 tbsp coriander leaves | ¼ tsp cumin seeds | 5 gm garlic | 50 gm chironji seeds | salt as per taste

Preparation method:

1. Soak chironji seeds and almonds for 4 hours.
2. Drain the water and grind chironji seeds and almonds without adding water.
3. Chop onion and coriander leaves, finely crush the garlic.
4. In a bowl, mix ground seeds, chopped onion, red chilli powder, cumin seeds, garlic and coriander leaves.
5. Divide into small balls and roll into a vada shape.
6. Heat coconut oil in a pan over low heat. Add the shaped vadas and fry on all sides until golden.
Serve warm with your favourite chutney.

Serving size (pieces/no)	Energy (Kcal)	Total Carbohydrate (gm)	Fibre (gm)	Fat (gm)	Protein (gm)
2 no	233	29.6	5	117	8.8

Masala Papad

Ingredients:

½ tbsp almond flour| 20g cucumber | ¼ cup onion | 2 tsp coriander leaves | 2 tsp lemon juice | ¼ tsp turmeric powder | ¼ cup tomato | ¼ cumin powder | 1/5 tbsp flaxseed powder | 2 tsp sesame seeds powder | ¼ cup mozzarella cheese | ¼ chaat masala | 2 tsp pumpkin | seeds powder | ½ tsp red chilli flakes

Preparation method:

1. Melt cheese in the microwave for 20 seconds.
2. In a bowl, mix almond flour, flaxseed powder, sesame seeds powder, pumpkin seeds powder, turmeric powder, cumin powder, red chilli flakes, salt and melted cheese. Knead to the consistency of a dough.
3. Divide the dough into two uniform balls. Place a dough ball between 2 parchment papers and roll into a thin, round shape.
4. Heat a non-stick pan over low heat, place the rolled papad dough and cook on both sides until crispy and golden brown.
5. Repeat the previous step with the remaining dough.
6. Garnish the papads with finely chopped onions, tomato, cucumber, coriander leaves and lemon juice.
7. Sprinkle chaat masala and serve.

Serving size (pieces/no)	Energy (Kcal)	Total Carbohydrate (gm)		Fibre (gm)	Fat (gm)	Protein (gm)
1 no	223.1	15.8		5.2	14.2	11.3

Pav Bhaji

Ingredients:

2 eggs | 5 tbsp unsalted butter | 50 g cauliflower| ¼ tsp turmeric powder | ½ carrot | ½ green bell pepper | 1 tomato | 3 beans | 1 tbsp butter | ½ cup almond flour| 1 onion | ½ tsp ginger garlic paste | ½ tsp red chilli powder| pav bhaji masala powder

Preparation method:

For Pav:
1. In an electric beater or hand beater add almond flour, egg, baking powder, 2 tbsp butter, salt to taste and beat for 10 minutes.
2. Grease a pan with butter and pour the batter. Bake the bun in an oven toaster grill at 230° C for 10 minutes and cut into 4 pieces.

For bhaji:
1. Pressure cook cauliflower, carrot, capsicum and beans for 2

whistles. Once pressure settles down, mash it with a spatula.

2. Add tomato in hot water. Peel the skin and mash the tomato.

3. Heat a pan with oil on medium heat, add ¼ onion, ginger garlic paste and sauté until fragrant.

4. Add tomato puree and sauté. Add red chilli powder, turmeric powder, pav bhaji masala, stevia, ½ tsp salt and mix well.

5. Lower the flame, add butter and mashed vegetables. Cook for 5-7 minutes, garnish with lemon juice and coriander leaves.

6. Heat another pan with butter on medium heat, slice the bun into two and toast on both sides.

7. Pav bhaji is ready to serve.

Serving size (pieces/no)	Energy (Kcal)	Total Carbohydrate (gm)	Fibre (gm)	Fat (gm)	Protein (gm)
4 no	244.51	9.89	3.842	37.9	6.3

Kachori

Ingredients:

¼ cup curd | ¼ cup broccoli | 2 tbsp coconut oil | ½ tsp xanthan gum | ½ cup coconut flour| ½ cup almond flour| 1 green chilli | ½ tsp garam masala powder | 2 tbsp coriander leaves | ½ tsp ajwain

Preparation method:

1. For the filling, grate broccoli and finely chop green chilli, coriander leaves and almonds.

2. Heat coconut oil in a pan over medium heat. Add broccoli, green chilli, coriander leaves, and salt.

3. Sauté for 2 minutes and allow to cool.

4. In a bowl, mix almond flour, coconut flour, xanthan gum, curd, ajwain, garam masala, ¼ tsp salt and water. Knead to the consistency of a roti dough.

5. Make small balls of the dough, cover and rest for 20-30 mins.

6. Divide the dough into small balls. Flatten the dough and place the stuffing inside to make a round ball, brush it with coconut oil.

7. Repeat the previous step with the remaining dough.

8. Preheat the oven to 180° C for 10 minutes and bake the kachori

on both sides for 15 minutes each.
9. Serve warm with your favourite chutney.

Serving size (pieces/no)	Energy (Kcal)	Total Carbohydrate (gm)	Fibre (gm)	Fat (gm)	Protein (gm)
1 no	106.375	7.575	4.08	8.05	3.125

Boiled peanut chaat

Ingredients:

30g boiled peanuts | 1 tsp lemon juice | 1 tbsp cucumber | 1 tbsp tomato | ½ tsp green chilli | 1 tsp coriander leaves | ¼ tsp red chilli powder | ¼ tsp chaat masala | salt for taste

Preparation method:

1. Boil peanuts in a pressure cooker with water and salt. Cook for 12-15 minutes. Drain off all the water and cool down for 5 minutes.
2. Chop all the vegetables in small pieces.
3. In a mixing bowl, add peanuts, cucumber, tomato, green chilli, coriander leaves, red chilli powder and chaat masala.
4. Toss all ingredients well so that the peanuts are well seasoned.
5. Boiled peanut chaat is ready to serve.

Serving size (gm/cup)	Energy (Kcal)	Total Carbohydrate (gm)	Fibre (gm)	Fat (gm)	Protein (gm)
1 cup (100 gm)	218	15.62	5.96	15.32	9.71

Chia pudding

Ingredients:

1 tbsp chia seeds | ½ cup almond milk | ½ fruit strawberry | nuts

Preparation method:

1. In a mason jar/ dessert bowl add the chia seeds.
2. Pour the milk/curd of your choice and stir well.
3. Cover it & let it sit for a minimum of 4 hours or overnight.
4. Once the chia seeds soak in & double up add chopped berries/strawberries
5. Garnish with nuts.

Other options

Use coconut milk or curd or yogurt instead of almond milk
Use any other berries instead of strawberries

Tip: Add or reduce the liquid content as per the consistency of one's choice.

Serving size (ml/cup)	Energy (Kcal)	Total Carbohydrate (gm)	Fibre (gm)	Fat (gm)	Protein (gm)
1 cup (100ml)	94	9.78	6.4	5.44	2.81

EGGETARIAN

Zucchini egg fried rice

Ingredients:

2 cup grated zucchini | 2 tbsp beans | 2 tbsp green peas | 2 tbsp capsicum | 2 eggs | 1 tbsp coconut aminos (sauce) | salt for taste | 1 tsp pepper | 1 tsp coconut oil

Preparation method:

1. Grate zucchini and chop the other vegetables.
2. Scramble the eggs with a pinch of salt and pepper.
3. In a pan, cook the vegetables with little water.
4. Sauté the zucchini in ghee or butter until soft.
5. Heat coconut oil in a pan, add vegetables, scrambled egg and mix well.
6. Add salt, pepper and coconut aminos.
7. Mix well and serve hot.

Other options

Sauce: use soya sauce or chilli sauce for spices
Garnish: Garnish with the spring onions and coriander leaves
Instead of zucchini use cauliflower, cabbage, bell pepper and broccoli

Serving size (gm/cup)	Energy (Kcal)	Total Carbohydrate (gm)	Fibre (gm)	Fat (gm)	Protein (gm)
1 cup (100gm)	151.3	12.97	3.8	6.14	10.47

Omelette stuffed bell peppers

Ingredients:

50 g onion | 50 g tomato | 2-3 tbsp spinach | ¼ tbsp pepper | 2 slices cheese | 2 capsicum | 2 eggs | Salt to taste | 1 tbsp butter | 1-2 tbsp mixed herbs

Preparation method:

1. Cut capsicum into thick circles. Grease a baking tray, and place the cut side of the green capsicum on the tray. Brush with butter and bake at 170° C for 10 min until both sides are partially cooked or microwave on medium for 10 minutes on both sides.
2. In a bowl, add onion, tomato, spinach, pepper, salt and eggs and beat well.
3. Pour the above mixture into the precooked capsicum (don't overfill).
4. Dress capsicum circles with shredded cheese and sprinkle herbs.
5. Bake the capsicum with egg mixture for 15 min at 170° C or until the cheese melts.
6. Flip on the other side to cook both sides.
7. If you don't have an oven or OTG, cut capsicum into circles, fill it with the egg mixture and cook in a flat pan by placing capsicum circles on a buttered pan, cover and cook on both sides for 10 min on low flame.

Other options

Herbs: cilantro, parsley, celery
Instead of egg use Paneer or tofu

Serving size (pieces/no)	Energy (Kcal)	Total Carbohydrate (gm)	Fibre (gm)	Fat (gm)	Protein (gm)
4 nos	437.47	22.14	6.2	28.3	27.36

Flaxseed & egg uttapam

Ingredients:

2 whole eggs | 4 tsp coconut oil | 1 tomato | half cup
chopped onions | 5 tbsp flaxseeds | 2 green chillies |
coriander leaves | salt to taste | ½ cup chopped onions |
2 tsp coriander leaves | 5 tbsp flaxseed powder

Preparation method:

1. In a bowl, mix the flaxseed powder, eggs, and salt.
2. Heat a tawa on a medium flame. Ladle out the batter and spread
it on the tawa.
3. Add onions, tomatoes, green chillies, and coriander leaves on top
of the batter.
4. Sprinkle coconut oil around the uttapam and cook it on both
sides.
5. Serve warm with vegetable chutney.

Other options

Garnish: add grated coconut kernels, grated cheese or paneer
Instead of onions use spring onions
Instead of normal tomato use cherry tomato

Serving size (pieces/no)	Energy (Kcal)	Total Carbohydrate (gm)	Fibre (gm)	Fat (gm)	Protein (gm)
2 no	250	8.48	3.67	18.37	15.7

Egg idli

Ingredients:

2 egg whites | 1/2 tsp baking soda | 1 tbsp curd | 1 tsp ghee
| 200g paneer |1 tbsp psyllium husk | 1/4 cup coconut flour|
salt to taste

Preparation method:

1. Put all the ingredients in a mixer grinder. Grind it to fine paste

(No need to add water).
2. Batter should be of thick consistency.
3. Apply ghee on an idli plate and place the batter in idli moulds.
4. Cook the idli for 5 to 8 mins.
5. Serve hot with sambhar or chutney.

Other options
Coconut idli without egg, idli with almond flour, idli with vegetable mix, paneer idli without egg

Serving size (pieces/no)	Energy (Kcal)	Total Carbohydrate (gm)	Fibre (gm)	Fat (gm)	Protein (gm)
4 no	288.07	5.743	1.67	20.24	20.66

Egg salad

Ingredients:
4 eggs | 1/2 tsp salt | 1/4 cup mayonnaise | 1/4 tsp black pepper powder | 1/4 cup fresh dill | 2 tbsp chive | 2 tbsp Dijon mustard

Preparation method:
1. Boil eggs in water and let stand for 10-12 minutes
2. Peel and chop the eggs and add them to a medium sized bowl.
3. Add mayonnaise, dill, chives, Dijon mustard, salt and pepper.
4. Mix well & enjoy your egg salad.

Other options
Egg salad with avocado, egg salad with lettuce wraps
Dressing: Avocado, cream, heavy whipping cream

Serving size (gm/cup)	Energy (Kcal)	Total Carbohydrate (gm)	Fibre (gm)	Fat (gm)	Protein (gm)
1 cup (100gm)	178.4	1.467	0.336	12.9	13.176

Mixed seed egg dosa

Ingredients:

2 whole eggs | 1/2 tsp natural sea salt | 1/2 tbsp cream | 1 tbsp raw sunflower seeds | 1 tbsp butter | 15 almonds | 5 dried red chilli | 3 tbsp watermelon seed | 4 garlic cloves | 1/4 tsp lemon juice | 3 tbsp flaxseed | 2 tbsp coconut oil

Preparation method:

1. Deseed the red chillies and soak in hot water for 15 minutes.
2. Grind the soaked red chillies into a smooth paste.
3. Heat unsalted butter in a pan on medium heat. Sauté chopped garlic for 2 minutes.
4. Add the chilli paste and a pinch of salt, and sauté until it reaches a thick consistency.
5. Turn off the heat and add lemon juice. Mix well and keep aside.
6. **For the batter** - Grind melon seeds, sunflower seeds, almonds, and flaxseeds to a fine powder. Mix with 1/2 cup of water to make a batter.
7. Whisk eggs in a bowl and mix it with the seed batter and salt.
8. Let the batter rest for 10 minutes.
9. Heat a non-stick tawa on medium flame. Ladle out the batter and spread it on the tawa. Sprinkle with ghee and cook the dosa on both sides.
10. Spread the dry chilli paste on top of the dosa.
11. Serve warm with chutney.

Other options

Almond egg dosa
Instead of egg use mozzarella cheese
Instead of water, add almond milk or coconut milk
Instead of coconut oil use ghee or butter

Serving size (pieces/no)	Energy (Kcal)	Total Carbohydrate (gm)	Fibre (gm)	Fat (gm)	Protein (gm)
2 no	432.07	9.6	4.8	35.84	21.93

Egg pancake

Ingredients:

2 whole eggs | 1/4 tsp salt | 1/2 cup coconut | 2 tbsp coconut oil

Preparation method:

1. Grind coconut into a fine paste.
2. Beat the eggs with salt and add to the coconut paste. Batter should be a thick consistency.
3. Heat a tawa on medium flame and add 1 teaspoon of coconut oil.
4. Scoop a portion of batter and spread it on the pan.
5. Cook the pancake on both sides.

Serving size (pieces/no)	Energy (Kcal)	Total Carbohydrate (gm)	Fibre (gm)	Fat (gm)	Protein (gm)
2 no	289	5.27	2.7	24.05	14

Egg noodles

Ingredients:

2 whole eggs | salt to taste | 2 tbsp unsalted butter | 50g paneer | 1 bell pepper | 1 tomato | 1 tbsp butter | 1 onion | 2 garlic cloves | 1 green chilli | 1/4 tsp red chilli powder | 1/4 tsp lemon juice | 1/2 tsp black pepper

Preparation method:

1. Chop onion, tomato, capsicum, and garlic into strips/ slices.
2. In a bowl, beat eggs with salt and chilli powder.
3. Heat butter in a pan and fry the egg. Cut the fried egg into thin strips to resemble noodles and keep it aside.
4. Heat 1 tbsp butter in a pan.
5. Cut paneer into strips, and sauté in the butter for 2 minutes. Remove the paneer and keep it aside.
6. In the same pan, add the remaining butter, onion, tomato, capsicum, and garlic, and sauté with a little salt.

7. Add green chilli, egg noodles, sautéed paneer, pepper powder, and lemon juice, and sauté for 2 minutes
Serve warm.

Other options

Egg noodle with cheese Keto egg noodles with chicken
Sauce: soya sauce, chilli sauce, tomato sauce
Herbs: parsley, basil, oregano
Instead of butter use coconut oil or ghee
Instead of paneer use tofu

Serving size (gm/cup)	Energy (Kcal)	Total Carbohydrate (gm)	Fibre (gm)	Fat (gm)	Protein (gm)
1 cup (100gm)	386.3	12.54	1.97	29.95	16.05

Egg paddu

Ingredients:

2 eggs | 2 tbsp coconut oil | 1 tbsp bell pepper | 1 tbsp onion | 1 dry chilli | 1 slice cheddar cheese | 1 green chilli | 1 tbsp coriander leaves | 100ml water | 1 tbsp sesame seed powder | salt to taste | 2 tbsp spring onions

Preparation method:

1. Finely Chop the onion, capsicum, green chilli, spring onion, and coriander leaves.
2. Heat coconut oil in a pan. Sauté the chopped vegetables for 2 minutes on medium heat.
3. Whisk the egg well with hand beater/ electric beater. Add chilli flakes and sautéed vegetables to the whisked egg mixture.
4. Add salt, grated cheese, and sesame seed powder to the egg mixture.
5. Heat the paddu vessel, add some oil, and pour the paddu mixture.
6. Cover and cook on both sides on low heat for 5 minutes.
7. Serve warm with chutney.

Other options

Egg paddu with paneer, Egg paddu with mushroom, Egg paddu with tofu, Egg paddu with leafy vegetables
Instead of coconut oil use ghee or butter

Serving size (pieces/no)	Energy (Kcal)	Total Carbohydrate (gm)	Fibre (gm)	Fat (gm)	Protein (gm)
4 no	401.1	13.43	2.8	29.2	25.96

NON-VEGETARIAN

Cauliflower chicken biryani

Ingredients:

100g whole milk plain yogurt | 2 tbsp butter | 1 whole clove | cinnamon stick |1 cardamom |1 bay leaf |1 tomato | 2 tbsp coconut oil |1/2 cup chopped onions | 2 tbsp ginger and garlic | 1½ cup cauliflower rice |1/4 tsp grounded dry chilli | 1/4 tsp lemon juice | 1 cup raw chicken | 1/4 tsp pepper | 10 mint leaves | 1/4 tbsp biriyani masala powder | green chilli | salt to taste.

Preparation method:

1. Marinate chicken with curd, 1/2 tbsp ginger- garlic paste and salt for 1 hour.
2. Heat 2 tbsp oil in a pan. Add chopped onions, sauté till onion becomes translucent.
3. Now add marinated chicken, pepper and cook till the gravy becomes semi dry. Keep it aside.
4. Heat a pan, add ghee and fry cinnamon, clove, cardamom and bay leaf.
5. Add the remaining ginger-garlic paste and sauté until raw smell goes.
6. Add tomato, mint, green chilli, chilli powder and biryani masala powder, and sauté for 10 mins in low flame.
7. Add the cauliflower rice, lemon juice and chicken gravy and mix. Cover with a lid.
8. Garnish with coriander leaves.
9. Serve hot with raita

Serving size (gm/cup)	Energy (Kcal)	Total Carbohydrate (gm)	Fibre (gm)	Fat (gm)	Protein (gm)
1 cup (100gm)	149.6	24.41	3.86	2.39	10.03

Chicken zucchini noodles

Ingredients:

2 tbsp butter | 3 Zucchini | black pepper powder to taste | 4 garlic cloves | 2 Chicken breasts (boneless, without skin) | 1/2 tsp red chilli flakes | Salt to taste

Preparation method:

1. Heat a large heavy-duty pan on medium/high heat.
2. Add butter and minced garlic to the pan.
3. Cook garlic for 30 seconds to 1 minute or until fragrant.
4. Add the chicken, red chilli flakes, salt and pepper.
5. Fry the chicken for 5-6 minutes or until golden and cooked thoroughly.
6. Toss in the zucchini noodles (zucchini that has been spiralized or cut into thin strips) and cook for 1 minute, then turn off the heat.
7. Sprinkle with cheese if desired.

For all non-vegetarian dishes, you may use chicken, fish, lamb, pork, crab, shrimp, prawns or eggs.

Other options

Spices: Ginger, garam masala
Herbs: Oregano, rosemary, parsley, celery, cilantro, lemon grass

For cooking chicken, instead of water use coconut milk
Instead of butter use coconut oil or ghee

Serving size (gm/cup)	Energy (Kcal)	Total Carbohydrate (gm)	Fibre (gm)	Fat (gm)	Protein (gm)
1 cup (100gm)	106	7.43	1.7	5.11	8.75

Pepper chicken

Ingredients:

2 cups chicken | 1 cup full fat greek yogurt | 50g butter | 2 tsp coconut oil | ½ tsp red chilli powder | salt for taste | 50g black pepper corns whole | 1 cup full fat greek yogurt

Preparation method:

1. Wash the chicken thoroughly and pat it dry.
2. Grind black pepper coarsely.
3. In a bowl, add curd, half of the ground black pepper, salt and red chilli powder.
4. Add the chicken and mix with your hands, until the chicken is fully seasoned.
5. Add coconut oil to the marinade, and mix well.
6. Let the chicken rest in the fridge for four to five hours.
7. Heat butter in a thick bottomed pan. Add the remaining ground black pepper.
8. Place the chicken in the butter and cook on low heat.
9. After 4-5 minutes, cover the chicken for 10-12 minutes on low heat. Keep stirring at regular intervals.
10. Once the chicken has an even golden colour, it is ready.
11. Serve hot.

Other options

Fried chicken, air fry chicken breast, oven fried chicken, fried chicken strips, crispy fried chicken

Serving size (gm/cup)	Energy (Kcal)	Total Carbohydrate (gm)	Fibre (gm)	Fat (gm)	Protein (gm)
1 cup (100gm)	184.14	1.19	0.642	6.2	14.142

Grilled chicken

Ingredients:

2 cup chicken legs with thigh and back meat | 2 tbsp greek yogurt | 2 tbsp coconut oil | ½ tbsp dried oregano | 2 tsp ginger and garlic paste | 2 tbsp vinegar | 1 green chilli | salt to taste

Preparation method:

1. Wash the chicken well and pat dry.
2. Use a fork to poke the chicken all over.
3. In a bowl mix all the ingredients well.
4. Now add the chicken pieces to the bowl, and apply the marinade all over.
5. Allow the chicken to sit in the marinade overnight or for at least 4-5 hours.
6. Place the chicken on the grill pan, cover it with the lid, and cook on low heat.
7. Cook on one side for 5-7 minutes and then flip it over.
8. The chicken will be ready in 15 minutes.
9. Eat the chicken by itself, or add vegetables of your choice to the marinade, and cook them with the chicken.
10. Serve warm.

Serving size (gm/cup)	Energy (Kcal)	Total Carbohydrate (gm)	Fibre (gm)	Fat (gm)	Protein (gm)
1 cup (100gm)	167	14.77	0.7	5.34	14.83

Fish fry

Ingredients:

2 cup fish | 1/3 cup besan flour| 1 tbsp red chilli powder | 1 tsp ginger paste | 1 tsp garlic paste | 1 tbsp lemon juice | 1 egg| 1 tsp chaat masala | 10 tbsp coconut oil| 2 lemon wedges | salt to taste

Preparation method:

1. Place a piece of fish in a bowl.
2. Add red chilli powder, ginger paste, garlic paste, lemon juice, salt and besan flour to the fish. Mix well keep it aside for half an hour
3. Heat the coconut oil sufficiently. Break an egg and beat it in a separate bowl. Dip the fish in egg and drop it in hot oil.
4. Fry the fish until it gets a golden crust on the outside.
5. Place them in a serving plate.
6. Before serving, sprinkle chaat masala and place lemon wedges beside it.

Serving size (gm/cup)	Energy (Kcal)	Total Carbohydrate (gm)	Fibre (gm)	Fat (gm)	Protein (gm)
1 cup (100gm)	218	11	1.8	9.66	21.44

Sautéed dried shrimps

Ingredients:

30 gm dried mini shrimp | 30 gm chopped onions | 2 tsp ghee | pinch of turmeric powder | ¼ tsp mustard seeds | ¼ tsp chilli powder| curry leaves| salt to taste

Preparation method:

1. Heat ghee in a pan and fry the curry leaves until they turn crispy.
2. Add mustard seeds. When it splutters, lower the heat, and add the fried curry leaves.
3. Add chopped onions, and sauté till they change translucent.
4. Add salt, turmeric, and red chilli powder. Sauté on low heat.
5. Drop the shrimps in the pan and lower the heat.
6. Now add a little water, cover, and cook for 3 - 4 minutes.
7. Serve warm.

Serving size (gm/cup)	Energy (Kcal)	Total Carbohydrate (gm)	Fibre (gm)	Fat (gm)	Protein (gm)
1 cup (100gm)	161.9	9.7	1.4	6.48	18.176

Grilled fish

Ingredients:

7-8 pieces fish steaks | 2 tsp coconut oil | 1 tsp lemon juice | 1 tsp red chilli powder | 1 tsp ginger garlic paste | pepper & salt to taste

Preparation method:

1. Combine coconut oil, lemon juice, ginger garlic paste, chilli powder, salt, and pepper together.
2. Place the fish pieces in a dish and pour the spice and oil mixture on it.
3. Cover the dish and refrigerate for 1 hour.
4. Heat the grill. Place the fish pieces on the grill.
5. Cook for 5 minutes on both sides until cooked.
6. Serve hot.

Serving size (gm/cup)	Energy (Kcal)	Total Carbohydrate (gm)	Fibre (gm)	Fat (gm)	Protein (gm)
1 cup (100gm)	126	5.08	1	5.33	14.57

Prawn fry

Ingredients:

1 cup prawns | 1 tsp turmeric powder | 1 tbsp ghee | ½ tsp mustard seeds | 5-10 curry leaves | ½ tsp red chilli powder | salt to taste

Preparation method:

1. Clean the prawns and apply turmeric powder on them. Keep them aside for 1-2 hours.
2. Heat ghee in a pan and add mustard seeds and curry leaves.
3. Remove water from the prawns and place them in the pan.
4. Add chilli powder and salt.
5. Fry the prawns for about 5 mins, until they are cooked properly.
6. Serve hot.

Serving size (gm/cup)	Energy (Kcal)	Total Carbohydrate (gm)	Fibre (gm)	Fat (gm)	Protein (gm)
1 cup (100gm)	130.2	5.67	1.01	6.29	13.25

NOTE: Nutritive values are calculated based on the ingredients mentioned in the respective recipes. However, values may vary depending on the number/ quantity consumed.

Diet plan 1: Vegetarian

Breakfast	Stir fried vegetable (1 bowl), Bullet coffee (1 cup), Scrambled paneer (1 bowl), Star fruit (1 no)
Lunch	Stir fried vegetables (1 bowl), curd (½ cup), Moong dosa (2 nos) + ridge gourd chutney (1 tbsp)
Dinner	Stir fried vegetable (1 bowl), cup Curd (½ cup), Cauliflower palak rice (1 ½ cup)

Nutritive value for each meal

	Energy (Kcal)	Total Carbohydrate (gm)	Fibre (gm)	Fat (gm)	Protein (gm)
Breakfast	281.72	25.44	5.63	16.3	14.26
Lunch	397.26	30.55	8.534	23.692	18.784
Dinner	240.87	18.25	5.3	14.26	13.91

Nutritive value per day

Energy (Kcal)	Total Carbohydrate (gm)	Fibre (gm)	Fat (gm)	Protein (gm)
919.85	74.243	19.464	54.252	46.955

Diet plan 2: Vegetarian

Breakfast	Stir fried vegetable (1 bowl), Bullet coffee (1 cup), Dhokla (3-4 nos) + mint chutney (1 tbsp)
Lunch	Avocado vegetable salad (1 bowl), Curd (1/2 cup), Cauliflower Bisibelebath (1 1/2 cup)
Dinner	Sautéed mushroom with cream (1 bowl), Curd (1/2 cup), Almond coconut uttapam (2 nos) + mint chutney (1 tbsp)

Nutritive value for each meal

	Energy (Kcal)	Total Carbohydrate (gm)	Fibre (gm)	Fat (gm)	Protein (gm)
Breakfast	336.62	26.55	7.831	23.85	9.725
Lunch	420.9	29.62	12.25	29.46	15.174
Dinner	498.6	22.787	7.225	37.77	21.49

Nutritive value per day

Energy (Kcal)	Total Carbohydrate (gm)	Fibre (gm)	Fat (gm)	Protein (gm)
1256.17	78.957	27.306	91.08	46.36

Diet plan 3: Vegetarian

Breakfast	Stir fried vegetable (1 bowl), Coconut coffee/ tea (1 cup), Mixed dal dosa (2 nos) + walnut chutney (1 tbsp)
Lunch	Stir fried vegetable with cheese (1 bowl), Curd (1/2 cup), Pumpkin pulao (1 1/2 cup)
Dinner	Broccoli stir fried with coconut (1 bowl), Curd (1/2 cup), Paneer paratha (1-2 no)+mint chutney (1 tbsp)

Nutritive value for each meal

	Energy (Kcal)	Total Carbohydrate (gm)	Fibre (gm)	Fat (gm)	Protein (gm)
Breakfast	428.77	49.96	19.86	45.168	17.564
Lunch	385.3	34.65	9.4	20.97	21.456
Dinner	572.4	43.627	109.27	26.09	43.659

Nutritive value per day

Energy (Kcal)	Total Carbohydrate (gm)	Fibre (gm)	Fat (gm)	Protein (gm)
1386.4	127.93	138.53	92.227	82.56

Diet plan 4: Vegetarian

Breakfast	Stir fried vegetable (1 bowl), Coconut coffee/ tea 1 cup, Coriander vadi (3-4 nos) + mint chutney (1 tbsp), Star fruit (1 no)
Lunch	Stir fried vegetable (1 bowl), Curd (1/2 cup), Amaranth leaves paratha(1-2 nos) + raita (1/2 cup)
Dinner	Stir fried vegetable (1 bowl), Curd (1/2 cup), Creamy mushroom soup (1 bowl), Cheese pizza (2-3 slices)

Nutritive value for each meal

	Energy (Kcal)	Total Carbohydrate (gm)	Fibre (gm)	Fat (gm)	Protein (gm)
Breakfast	595.2	40.37	16.995	45.09	14.67
Lunch	739.1	43.76	14.25	34.57	34.29
Dinner	638.7	23.51	6.479	52.36	22.26

Nutritive value per day

Energy (Kcal)	Total Carbohydrate (gm)	Fibre (gm)	Fat (gm)	Protein (gm)
1973.05	107.64	37.72	132.02	71.22

Diet plan 5: Vegetarian

Breakfast	Stir fried vegetable (1 bowl), Coconut shake (1 1/2 cup), Star fruit (1 no)
Lunch	Stir fried vegetable (1 bowl), Curd (1/2 cup), Coconut roti (2 nos) + palak paneer (1.0 bowl)
Dinner	Zucchini salad (1 bowl),Curd (1/2 cup), Cauliflower curd rice (1 1/2 Cup)

Nutritive value for each meal

	Energy (Kcal)	Total Carbohydrate (gm)	Fibre (gm)	Fat (gm)	Protein (gm)
Breakfast	340.5	19.11	8.58	26.59	10.31
Lunch	590	50.37	10.91	30.06	33.04
Dinner	566.25	14.14	5.9	22.085	19.68

Nutritive value per day

Energy (Kcal)	Total Carbohydrate (gm)	Fibre (gm)	Fat (gm)	Protein (gm)
1496.7	83.62	25.39	78.7	63.02

Diet plan 6: Vegetarian

Breakfast	Stir fried vegetable (1 bowl), Bullet coffee (1 cup), Cauliflower poha (1 1/2 bowl)
Lunch	Mushroom sauteed (1 bowl), Curd (1/2 cup), Spinach soup with cream (1 bowl)
Dinner	Avocado salad (1 bowl), Curd (1/2 cup), Cauliflower paratha (1/2 no) + mint chutney (1 tbsp)

Nutritive value for each meal

	Energy (Kcal)	Total Carbohydrate (gm)	Fibre (gm)	Fat (gm)	Protein (gm)
Breakfast	422.3	28.49	7.9	34.53	12.32
Lunch	433.8	18.21	5.89	25.95	17.57
Dinner	584.95	46.78	8.15	29.588	19.889

Nutritive value per day

Energy (Kcal)	Total Carbohydrate (gm)	Fibre (gm)	Fat (gm)	Protein (gm)
1441	93.48	21.94	90.06	49.77

Diet plan 7: Vegetarian

Breakfast	Stir fried vegetable (1 bowl), Amla juice, Coconut uttapam (2 nos) + ridge gourd chutney (1 tbsp)
Lunch	Strawberry salad (1 bowl), 1/2 cup raita, Cauliflower fried rice (1 1/2 cup)
Dinner	Stir fried vegetable (1 bowl), 1/2 cup curd, seeds and nuts chapatti (2 nos)+ palak panner (1 cup)

Nutritive value for each meal

	Energy (Kcal)	Total Carbohydrate (gm)	Fibre (gm)	Fat (gm)	Protein (gm)
Breakfast	500.4	26.87	11.86	41.54	9.85
Lunch	351	24.54	8.042	22.402	17.578
Dinner	476.2	26.29	15.319	26.74	19.619

Nutritive value per day

Energy (Kcal)	Total Carbohydrate (gm)	Fibre (gm)	Fat (gm)	Protein (gm)
1327.6	77.7	35.221	90.682	47.047

Diet plan 1: Non–vegetarian

Breakfast	Bullet proof coffee (1 cup), Stir fried veggies salad (1 bowl), Egg omelette with mushroom and cheese (1-2 nos)
Lunch	Chicken salad (1 bowl), 1⁄2 cup Curd, Cauliflower chicken rice (1 1⁄2 cup)
Dinner	Stir fried vegetable (1 bowl), Chicken soup (1 bowl), Butter chicken (100 gm) + coconut roti (2 nos)

Nutritive value for each meal

	Energy (Kcal)	Total Carbohydrate (gm)	Fibre (gm)	Fat (gm)	Protein (gm)
Breakfast	430.52	15.3	2.9	31.63	25.12
Lunch	407.4	45.64	7.09	10.625	35.425
Dinner	569.3	50.79	10.71	28.42	31.33

Nutritive value per day

Energy (Kcal)	Total Carbohydrate (gm)	Fiber (gm)	Fat (gm)	Protein (gm)
1407.2	111.56	20.7	70.675	91.875

Diet plan 2: Non–vegetarian

Breakfast	Bullet proof coffee, Boiled egg (4 nos), Stir fried veggies (1 bowl)
Lunch	Scrambled egg with broccoli and heavy cream (1 bowl), Mushroom creamy soup (1 bowl), Star fruit (1 no)
Dinner	Chicken veggies salad (1 bowl), Fish fry (150 gm), Optional: 1/2 cup Curd

Nutritive value for each meal

	Energy (Kcal)	Total Carbohydrate (gm)	Fibre (gm)	Fat (gm)	Protein (gm)
Breakfast	194.52	11.33	2.2	14.63	9.12
Lunch	527.6	18.85	7.595	40.08	24.06
Dinner	460	23.81	4	19.43	46.66

Nutritive value per day

Energy (Kcal)	Total Carbohydrate (gm)	Fibre (gm)	Fat (gm)	Protein (gm)
1185.1	53.9	13.7	74.14	79.84

272

Diet plan 3: Non–vegetarian

Breakfast	Bullet proof coffee (1 cup), Scrambled egg with veggies (1 bowl), Stir fried veggies (1 bowl)
Lunch	Stir fried vegetable (1 bowl), Curd (1/2 cup), Cauliflower chicken fried rice (1 1/2 cup)
Dinner	Egg salad (100 gm), Egg parotha (1-2 no) + mint chutney

Nutritive value for each meal

	Energy (Kcal)	Total Carbohydrate (gm)	Fibre (gm)	Fat (gm)	Protein (gm)
Breakfast	335.5	37.7	7.2	19.63	26.12
Lunch	390.6	25.93	8.3	18.99	32.68
Dinner	507.75	34.43	4.395	34.83	15.999

Nutritive value per day

Energy (Kcal)	Total Carbohydrate (gm)	Fibre (gm)	Fat (gm)	Protein (gm)
1233.8	60.36	19.8	73.45	74.79

Diet plan 4: Non–vegetarian

Breakfast	Bullet proof coffee (1 cup), Spinach egg omelette with lot of cheese (1 bowl), Stir fried veggies (1.0 bowl)
Lunch	Palak soup with cream (1 bowl), Chicken zucchini noodles (1 1/2 cup), Curd (1/2 cup)
Dinner	Baked spinach with cheese and cream (1 bowl), Grilled chicken (150 gm), Optional: 1/2 cup Curd

Nutritive value for each meal

	Energy (Kcal)	Total Carbohydrate (gm)	Fibre (gm)	Fat (gm)	Protein (gm)
Breakfast	498.5	14.05	3.2	37.63	31.12
Lunch	382.8	19.41	5.79	17.511	21.44
Dinner	388.5	32.855	2.65	15.45	29.89

Nutritive value per day

Energy (Kcal)	Total Carbohydrate (gm)	Fibre (gm)	Fat (gm)	Protein (gm)
1269.8	66.31	11.63	70.951	82.45

Diet plan 5: Non–vegetarian

Breakfast	Bullet proof coffee (1 cup), Fluffy egg with cheese (100 gm), Stir fried veggies (1.0 bowl)
Lunch	Creamy salmon soup (1 bowl), Grilled chicken (150 gm) + mint chutney (1 tbsp), Optional: Curd (1/2 cup)
Dinner	Stir fried veggies with cheese (1 bowl), Curd (1/2 cup), Egg paratha (1-2 nos) + mint chutney (1 tbsp)

Nutritive value for each meal

	Energy (Kcal)	Total Carbohydrate (gm)	Fibre (gm)	Fat (gm)	Protein (gm)
Breakfast	359.3	21.38	9.4	45.82	20.02
Lunch	354.5	24.73	1.05	13.1	33.515
Dinner	308.25	46.527	16.395	42.48	17.80

Nutritive value per day

Energy (Kcal)	Total Carbohydrate (gm)	Fiber (gm)	Fat (gm)	Protein (gm)
1102.05	92.637	26.845	101.40	71.33

Diet plan 6: Non–vegetarian

Breakfast	Bullet proof coffee (1 cup), Avocado smoothie (1 1⁄2 cup), Stir fried veggies (1 bowl)
Lunch	Sautéed dry shrimp (1 bowl), Butter chicken (100gm) + seeds roti (2. Nos), Stir fried veggies (1/2 bowl), Optional: Curd (1⁄2 cup)
Dinner	Creamy mushroom soup (1 bowl), Grilled fish (150 gm), Stir fried vegetable (1 bowl)

Nutritive value for each meal

	Energy (Kcal)	Total Carbohydrate (gm)	Fibre (gm)	Fat (gm)	Protein (gm)
Breakfast	327.52	27.41	5.2	21.23	13.28
Lunch	701.19	34.53	16.21	37.61	44.285
Dinner	517.8	18.32	4.115	40.22	22.15

Nutritive value per day

Energy (Kcal)	Total Carbohydrate (gm)	Fibre (gm)	Fat (gm)	Protein (gm)
1546.5	80.26	25.525	99.06	79.715

Diet plan 7: Non–vegetarian

Breakfast	Bullet proof coffee (1 cup), Egg pancake (2-3 nos), Stir fried veggies (1 bowl)
Lunch	Broccoli stir fried veggies (1 bowl), Zucchini egg noodles (1 1/2 cup), Curd (1/2 cup)
Dinner	Chicken salad (1 bowl), Prawn fry (150 gm), Chilli chicken (100 gm) + low carb high protein roti (2.0 no)

Nutritive value for each meal

	Energy (Kcal)	Total Carbohydrate (gm)	Fibre (gm)	Fat (gm)	Protein (gm)
Breakfast	181.524	20.05	2.6	10.73	7.42
Lunch	405	34.72	6.3	32.5	16.68
Dinner	687.8	28.03	14.871	25.146	45.511

Nutritive value per day

Energy (Kcal)	Total Carbohydrate (gm)	Fibre (gm)	Fat (gm)	Protein (gm)
1274.3	82.8	23.77	68.3	69.611

How to prepare Low carb flour at home:

1. Coconut flour:

Ingredients:
1 whole tender coconut.

Preparation method:
- Take a well matured coconut. Break the coconut and remove the water from it.
- Cut out the coconut pulp/flesh through knife. Separate the coconut pulp from hard shell.
- Peel off the brown skin from the white coconut pulp.
- Cut all the coconut pulp into small pieces and transfer into the blender.
- Add hot water to a blender and blend it into fine smooth paste.
- Let it cool for about 5 minutes.
- Strain the coconut milk through a muslin cloth or strainer. Remove all the milk from coconut.
- Squeeze out all the milk from the pulp.
- Preheat the oven to 170 °F. If oven not available, go for shade dry or sun dry.
- Spread the strained coconut pulp over the butter paper for oven drying.
- Use cotton cloth or muslin cloth for natural drying by spreading into a flat even layer for 4 days.
- If coconut pulp is large size break up into small pieces.
- Bake the pulp for 45 minutes.
- Transfer the dehydrated pulp to a food processor.
- Blend the coconut for 1- 2 minutes until it is finely ground.
- Store the flour in airtight container for future use as and when required.

2. Peanut flour:

Ingredients:
1 cup unsalted peanut or raw shelled peanuts.

Preparation method:
- Roast peanuts over a medium heat on a dry pan until they are slightly golden and smells really good.
- Let them cool down completely.
- Remove from the heat and spread them on a plate and let them cool down completely before blending.
- Please make sure that peanuts seeds are dry. Then add them to a blender.
- Turn the blender and blend for 5 seconds and stop the blender.
- Use a spoon to loosen the sticking flour at the bottom and sides of the blender.
- Make sure nothing sticks there. Then again start blending, repeat the step until it comes to fine powder consistency.
- Remove from the blender and transfer to a container. Don't close the lid let it cool down for 5 minutes.
- Then close the lid and you can store it in an ait tight container and keep them in the fridge for up to 3 months for future use as and when required.

3. Mixed seeds flour:

Ingredients:
- Peanut seeds- 500gm
- Coconut flour-500gm
- Soya flour- 500gm
- Besan flour- 200gm
- Almond nuts - 200 gm

- Sunflower seeds-100gm
- Pumpkin seeds-100gm
- Sesame seeds-50gm
- Isabgol/ psyllium husk-3 tbsp
- Karela seeds-100gm
- Methi seeds:100gm
- Xanthan gum- 3 tbsp.

Preparation method:
- Roast all the above seeds over a medium heat on a dry pan until they are slightly golden and smells really good.
- Remove from the heat and spread them out on a pan and let them cool down completely before blending.
- Please make sure that all the seeds are dry.
- Then add the xanthan gum to blender and blend it till fine powder.
- Add all the ingredients together into a blender and blend for 5 seconds.
- Use a spoon to loosen the sticking flour at the bottom and sides of the blender. Make sure nothing sticks there.
- Then again start blending repeat the step until it becomes fine powder consistency.
- Remove from the blender and transfer to a container. Don't close the lid let it cool down for 5 minutes.
- Then close the lid and you can store it in an air tight container and keep them in the fridge for future use up to 1-2 months

4. Low carb flour:

Ingredients:
- Buckwheat flour: 200gm
- Soya flour: 500gm

- Coconut flour: 500gm
- Sunflower: 500gm
- Flax seeds: 100gm
- Melon seeds: 100gm
- Pumpkin seeds: 100gm
- Karela seeds: 100gm
- Methi seeds: 100gm

Preparation method:
- Roast all the above ingredients over a medium heat on a dry pan until they are slightly golden and smells really good.
- Let them cool down completely.
- Remove from the heat and spread them out on a pan and let them cool down completely before blending.
- Please make sure that all the seeds are dry.
- Add all the ingredients together into blender. Turn the blender and blend for 5 seconds and stop the blender.
- Use a spoon to loosen the sticking flour at the bottom sides of the blender. Make sure nothing sticks there.
- Then again start blending repeat the step until it comes to a fine powder consistency.
- Remove from the blender and transfer to a container. Don't close the lid let it cool down for 5 minutes.
- Then close the lid and you can store it in an air tight container and keep them in the fridge for future use up to 1-2 months.

5. Almond flour:

Ingredients:
1 cup of raw or unsalted almonds.

Preparation method:

- Add almonds to a food processor or blender
- Turn the blender and blend for 5 seconds and stop the blender. Use a spoon to loosen the sticking flour at the bottom and sides of the blender. Make sure nothing is stuck there.
- Then again start blending repeat the step until it comes to a fine powder consistency.
- Remove from the blender and transfer to a container. Don't close the lid, let it cool down for 5 minutes.
- Store the flour in an air tight container at room temperature or in the fridge for future use.

How to prepare vegetable rice?

Cauliflower rice:

- Wash a cauliflower properly before using it. Then soak it in cooking vinegar for 30 minutes. After that, wash it in running water thoroughly. Take out the leaves from it.
- Separate the cauliflower florets from the stalks.
- Cut the stalk into cubes (similar to potato cubes)
- Take the stalk and grate it by a manual grater or blend it in a blender for 2 seconds till it comes to granular/ raw consistency.
- This granular cauliflower can be used in the form of rice and rawa.

With this you can prepare **curd rice, upma, poha, bisi bele bhath, khichdi, pongal, fried rice, coloured rice, pulao, biryani, etc.**

In the same way, you can also use other vegetables **cabbage/ zucchini/ broccoli** for making vegetable rice.

Tips for managing healthy sugars:

1. Start each meal (breakfast, lunch and dinner) with 1 bowl of stir-fried vegetables or rich fat salad with olive oil. Note 50-60% of your each meal should be vegetables.
2. Instead of normal flour use low carb flour options.
3. Instead of normal rice use vegetable rice (cauliflower/cabbage/broccoli/zucchini)
4. For a healthy gut add curd/yogurt in each meal.
5. Use mixed nuts and seeds for the snacks options anytime of the day (no dry fruits).
6. Drink 2-3ltrs of water per day.
7. Use cold pressed oils only. No refined vegetable seeds oil.
8. Reduce frequency of eating and take 2-3 meals only in a day.
9. Eat only when you are hungry.
10. Fruits: Avocado (Butter fruit), and the following fruits in moderation:
Guava, Musambi, Strawberry, Blueberry, Raspberry, Mulberry, Blackberry, Gooseberry (Amla), Star fruit, Palm fruit (Ice apple), Wood apple, Jamun fruit, Lemon.
Avoid all other fruits.
11. Avoid starchy foods, bakery items and all processed foods.
12. Physical activities should be done for about 30- 45 minutes a day, at least 5 days a week.
13. Follow the plate concept for each meal.

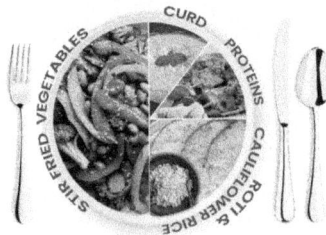

TABLE OF FIGURES

REFERENCES AND FURTHER READING

1. A fat lot of good - Dr. Peter Brukner
2. Always Hungry? By Dr. David Ludwing
3. Eat rich, live long by Ivor Cummins and Dr. Jeff Gerber
4. Get Strong by Al Kavadlo and Danny Kavadlo
5. Good calories, Bad calories by Gary Taubes
6. https://eatplaythrive.com.au/nutrition/
7. https://lowcarbdownunder.com.au/resources/
8. https://phcuk.org/sugar/
9. https://www.youtube.com/c/jerryteixeira
10. https://www.youtube.com/watch?v=wBsnk2PtPeo
11. Protein power by Michael and Mary Dan Eades
12. The Alzheimer's antidote by Amy Berger
13. The Art and Science of low carbohydrate living by Jeff Volek and Stephen Phinney
14. The big fat surprise by Nina Teicholz
15. The Diabetes code and the obesity code by Dr. Jason Fung
16. The Diabetes Solution by Dr. Richard Bernstein
17. The Hungry Brain by Stephan Guyenet
18. Why we get sick by Benjamin Bikman
19. www.dietdoctor.com/
20. www.ruled.me
21. www.youtube.com/watch?v=da1vvigy5tQ&feature=share
22. www.youtube.com/watch?v=Ekqq6DE8vGE
23. www.youtube.com/watch?v=Z

ABOUT THE AUTHOR

Dr. Bhujang Shetty was one of India's leading luminaries in the field of Ophthalmic Health Care. He founded Narayana Nethralaya in Bangalore over 40 years ago, which has been consistently named as one of the top 10 tertiary eye-care centers in India today. Having completed his MBBS degree in 1978, Dr. Shetty completed his ophthalmology training at Minto Ophthalmic Hospital - Bangalore Medical College in 1982.

In 2018, Dr. Shetty bagged the 'Legend in Ophthalmology' award at the Times Healthcare Achievers Award, while his institute, Narayana Nethralaya, was awarded the 'Best Ophthalmology Hospital.' He has been conferred the "Kannada Rajyotsava Award" for his yeomen services in the field of ophthalmology. Dr. Bhujang Shetty was the founder President of the Bangalore Ophthalmic Society.

Dr. Shetty penned the current book 'Diabetic No More' based on his personal experience of dealing with lifestyle diseases. He has explained in detail the various methods he embraced to get his life back on track after he was diagnosed with diabetes at the age of 40.